CAROLINAS MAP KEY

Other titles in this series

The Best in Tent Camping: Arizona
The Best in Tent Camping: Colorado
The Best in Tent Camping: Florida
The Best in Tent Camping: Georgia
The Best in Tent Camping: Illinois
The Best in Tent Camping: Kentucky
The Best in Tent Camping: Maryland
The Best in Tent Camping: Minnesota
The Best in Tent Camping: Missouri and the Ozarks
The Best in Tent Camping: Montana
The Best in Tent Camping: New England
The Best in Tent Camping: New Jersey
The Best in Tent Camping: New Mexico
The Best in Tent Camping: New York State
The Best in Tent Camping: Northern California
The Best in Tent Camping: Oregon
The Best in Tent Camping: Pennsylvania
The Best in Tent Camping: The Southern Appalachian and Smoky Mountains
The Best in Tent Camping: Southern California
The Best in Tent Camping: Tennessee
The Best in Tent Camping: Utah
The Best in Tent Camping: Virginia
The Best in Tent Camping: Washington
The Best in Tent Camping: West Virginia
The Best in Tent Camping: Wisconsin

For other books by Johnny Molloy, visit
johnnymolloy.com

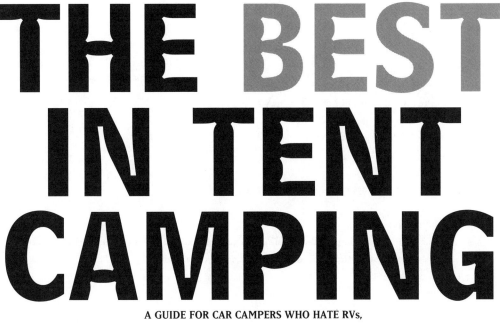

THE BEST IN TENT CAMPING

A GUIDE FOR CAR CAMPERS WHO HATE RVs,
CONCRETE SLABS, AND LOUD PORTABLE STEREOS

THE CAROLINAS

THIRD EDITION

JOHNNY MOLLOY

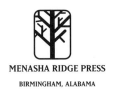

MENASHA RIDGE PRESS
BIRMINGHAM, ALABAMA

This book is for residents of North Carolina and South Carolina who enjoy some great places to live, work, and tent camp.

Published by Menasha Ridge Press

Distributed by Publishers Group West

Third edition, first printing

Library of Congress Cataloging-in-Publication Data

Molloy, Johnny, 1961-

 The best in tent camping the Carolinas : a guide for car campers who hate RVs, concrete slabs, and loud portable stereos / Johnny Molloy. -- 3rd ed.

 p. cm.

Includes index.

 ISBN-13: 978-0-89732-798-5

 ISBN-10: 0-89732-798-5

 1. Camping--North Carolina--Guidebooks. 2. Camp sites, facilities, etc.--North Carolina--Guidebooks. 3. North Carolina--Guidebooks. 4. Camping--South Carolina--Guidebooks. 5. Camp sites, facilities, etc.--South Carolina--Guidebooks. 6. South Carolina--Guidebooks. I. Title.

GV191.42.N2M65 2010

917.5068--dc22

2010017751

Cover and text design by Ian Szymkowiak, Palace Press International, Inc.

Cover photo © Steve Murray/Alamy: Brightly colored sky at sunrise over the Blue Ridge Mountains in North Carolina.

Author photo by Pam Morgan

Maps by Steve Jones and Johnny Molloy

Indexing by Jan Mucciarone

Menasha Ridge Press

P.O. Box 43673

Birmingham, Alabama 35243

www.menasharidge.com

THE BEST
IN TENT
CAMPING
CAROLINAS

TABLE OF CONTENTS

NORTH CAROLINA MOUNTAINS 7

NORTH CAROLINA PIEDMONT 69

NORTH CAROLINA COAST AND COASTAL PLAIN 89

SOUTH CAROLINA UPCOUNTRY 117

SOUTH CAROLINA MIDLANDS 139

SOUTH CAROLINA LOW COUNTRY 171

APPENDIXES AND INDEX 181

ACKNOWLEDGMENTS

I WOULD LIKE TO THANK ALL OF THE LAND MANAGERS of North Carolina's and South Carolina's state parks and forests, as well as the folks at the national forests, for helping me in the research and writing of this book.

Thanks to Aaron Marable for hiking with me on the Buncombe Trail, to Cisco Meyer for camping with me at Oconee State Park, to Lisa Daniel for camping with me on the South Carolina Coast, and to Steve Grayson and John Bland for going to the Tennessee–South Carolina football game in Columbia. Thanks to Linda Grebe at Eureka! for providing me with great tents both big and small. Thanks to Silva for their compasses and to Camp Trails for their packs. Thanks to travelin' Jean Cobb at Freebairn & Co. for her help. Thanks to Merrell for providing me great hiking shoes, to Lafuma for great packs and sleeping bags, and to Delorme for providing a quality GPS. Thanks to all the people involved with my writing of *50 Hikes in South Carolina*.

My biggest thanks of all goes to the people of North Carolina and South Carolina. They have beautiful and historic states in which to tent camp.

PREFACE

BEING A SOUTHERNER, I jumped at the opportunity to write *The Best in Tent Camping: The Carolinas.* And for the third edition, I jumped at the chance to update the great campgrounds in these great states. Having extensively explored the outdoors and written about North and South Carolina, I looked at writing this book as an opportunity to thoroughly and systematically explore the entirety of the two states, via tent camping of course. With a Eureka! tent and laptop computer in my Jeep, combined with my past experiences, I took off, exploring by day and tent camping at night, breaking out the computer to type up on-site reports about each destination.

My high expectations were exceeded. I knew the islands and beaches were beautiful from past visits, but have you been to the Outer Banks in fall, with a cool breeze and warm golden light spilling onto its sands? Have you explored the rich, forested interior of Hunting Island, then looked out from atop its lighthouse? To me, what lay between the Atlantic beaches and the Appalachian range was most surprising.

In North Carolina, Merchants Millpond State Park features a swamp not unlike the famed Okefenokee Swamp of Georgia. The Lumber River also has dark water and is a federally designated Wild and Scenic River. The Piedmont has the Uwharrie National Forest, where hiking trails wind beneath verdant forested hills broken by clear streams. Pilot Mountain stands where the Piedmont meets the hills, and its cylindrical, flat-topped cone rises 1,400 feet above the surrounding landscape.

In South Carolina, the pleasant surprises start in the Francis Marion National Forest, just a few miles inland from the Atlantic Ocean. This locale offers a long stretch of the Palmetto Trail, a nature study amid wooded wetlands, and canoe routes through some of the least-trammeled terrain in the Palmetto State. Sand Hills State Forest harbors an eco-system unique to the Carolinas. The varied tracts of the Sumter National Forest in the Midlands offer great recreational opportunities. The Buncombe Trail, now a South Carolina favorite of mine, circles sleepy Brick House Campground. Lick Fork Lake is an ideal mix of campground and land- and water-based recreation in an attractive setting. Leroy's Ferry Campground, operated by the U.S. Army Corps of Engineers, is a quiet respite on big Thurmond Lake. And Poinsett State Park is an ecological wonder, with vegetation from the sand hills, the mountains, and the coast, all in one great destination.

Even the mountains offered some new surprises, such as the New River in the north-west corner of North Carolina. This ancient watercourse winds its way through steep hills, offering excellent canoeing and fishing for smallmouth bass. For forays onto the river, use the Wagoner Unit of New River State Park as a base camp. The walk-in tent-camping sites at South Carolina's Oconee State Park make for shaded hideaways between walking treks on the Foothills Trail and the nearby paths it intersects.

With the aid of the helpful folks at Menasha Ridge Press, this third edition complete with updates has now come to be. I made many wonderful memories along the way and expect to make many more in the Carolinas. I hope this book will help you make some memories of your own.

—Johnny Molloy

THE BEST CAROLINAS CAMPGROUNDS

THE BEST
IN TENT
CAMPING

A GUIDE FOR CAR CAMPERS WHO HATE RVs,
CONCRETE SLABS, AND LOUD PORTABLE STEREOS

THE CAROLINAS

THIRD EDITION

INTRODUCTION

IT IS A PLEASURE to introduce the third edition of this book. North and South Carolina offer varied and scenic ecosystems, as well as a rich human history. Both states stretch from the alluring Blue Ridge Mountains in the west—the highest, and some would argue, the most scenic range of the Appalachians—to the saltwater-washed sands of the Atlantic coast in the east. The Southern Appalachians, unmatched in biodiversity amid temperate climes, offer shady forests through which clear streams dance over gray boulders, feeding rivers that race toward the Piedmont. Here, where the hills soften, the beauty is more subtle yet clearly alive to the discerning camper. Enhancing this natural charm, many rivers have been impounded to offer the tent camper endless water-recreation opportunities. The central lands give way to the coastal plain, where dark rivers quietly flow among brooding cypress trees. Moving east, the water of the mountains meets the water of the sea, forming rich estuarine habitats that further complement the ecosystem. Finally, the land ends at the Atlantic Ocean's edge, bordered by slender sand-island chains and shell-dotted beaches.

It is in the Carolinas where much of our country's formative history took place. For starters, did you know that more Revolutionary War battles between the Americans and the British took place in South Carolina than in any other state, or that the first English-speaking colonies in North America were in North Carolina? In fact, under a charter from Queen Elizabeth, Sir Walter Raleigh initiated two North Carolina colonies in the 1580s. It is this melding of human and natural history that makes exploring the Carolinas so appealing.

Today, tent campers can enjoy each of these distinct regions of the Carolinas. At the lofty altitude of 6,320 feet in Mount Mitchell State Park, you can pitch your tent at the highest campground in the East. Or camp along a federally designated Wild and Scenic River, such as the Chattooga or the New. The central Carolinas have quiet Woods Ferry, where Civil War soldiers once crossed the Broad River and where you can rejoin nature at West Morris Mountain. The coastal plain also has scenic rivers ready to be explored, such as the Lumber and the Little Pee Dee. A tent camper has to take a ferry to reach Ocracoke Campground. And there is Frisco Campground, about as far east as you can tent camp in the Carolinas, where tall dunes of sand rise high. All this spells paradise for the tent camper. No matter where you go, the scenery never fails to please the eye.

Before embarking on a trip, take time to prepare. Many of the best tent campgrounds are a fair distance from the civilized world, and you'll want to enjoy yourself rather than make supply or gear runs. Call ahead and ask for a park map, brochure, or other information to help you plan your trip. Visit campground Web sites for more information. Make reservations wherever applicable, especially at popular state parks. North Carolina state park campsites now take reservations! And don't forget to inquire about the latest reservation and entrance fees at state parks and forests.

Ask questions. Ask more questions. Although this guidebook is an indispensable tool for the Carolina-bound tent camper, the more questions you ask, the fewer surprises you will get. There are other times, however, when you'll grab your gear and this book, hop in the car, and just wing it. This can be an adventure in its own right.

THE RATING SYSTEM

Included in this book is a rating system for the Carolinas' best tent campgrounds. Certain attributes—beauty, site privacy, site spaciousness, quiet, security, and cleanliness and upkeep—are ranked using a star system. Five stars are ideal; one is acceptable. This system will help you find the campground that has the attributes you desire.

BEAUTY In the best campgrounds, the fluid shapes and elements of nature—flora, water, land, and sky—meld to create locales that seem tailor-made for tent camping. The best sites are so attractive that you may be tempted not to leave your outdoor home. A little campsite enhancement is necessary to make the scenic area camper-friendly, but too many reminders of civilization eliminated many a campground from inclusion in this book.

SITE PRIVACY A little understory foliage goes a long way in making you feel comfortable once you've picked your site for the night. Fortunately, there is a trend toward planting natural borders between campsites if the borders don't already exist. With some trees or brush to define the sites, campers have their own personal space. Then you can go about the pleasures of tent camping without keeping up with the Joneses at the site next door—or them with you.

SITE SPACIOUSNESS This attribute can be very important, depending on how much of a gearhead you are and the size of your group. Campers with family-style tents and screen shelters need a large, flat spot on which to pitch their tent, and they still have to get to the ice chest to prepare foods, all the while not getting burned near the fire ring. Gearheads need adequate space to show off their portable glow-in-the-dark lounge chairs and other pricey gewgaws to neighbors strolling by. I just want enough room to keep my bedroom, den, and kitchen separate.

QUIET The music of the lakes, rivers, and all the land between—singing birds, rushing streams, waves lapping against the shoreline, wind whooshing through the trees—includes the kinds of noises tent campers associate with being in the Carolinas. In concert, the sounds of nature camouflage the sounds you don't want to hear, such as autos coming and going or loud neighbors.

SECURITY Campground security is relative. A remote campground in an undeveloped area is usually safe, but don't tempt potential thieves by leaving your valuables out for all to see. Use common sense and go with your instincts. Campground hosts are wonderful to have around, and state parks with locked gates are ideal for security. Get to know your neighbors and develop a buddy system to watch each other's belongings when possible.

CLEANLINESS AND UPKEEP I'm a stickler for this one. Nothing sabotages a scenic campground like trash. Most of the campgrounds in this guidebook are clean. More-rustic campgrounds (my favorites) usually receive less maintenance. Busy weekends and holidays will show the effects; however, don't let a little litter spoil your good time. Help clean up, and think of it as doing your part for the Carolinas' natural environment.

THE OVERVIEW MAP AND KEY

Use the overview maps on the inside front and back covers to assess the exact location of each campground. The campground's number appears not only on the overview maps but also on the map key facing the overview map, in the table of contents, and on the profile's first page.

The book is organized by region, as indicated in the table of contents. A map legend that details the symbols found on the campground-layout maps appears on page 194.

CAMPGROUND-LAYOUT MAPS

Each profile contains a detailed campground-layout map that provides an overhead look at campground sites, internal roads, facilities, and other key items. Each campground entrance's GPS coordinates are included with each profile.

CAMPGROUND-ENTRANCE GPS COORDINATES

To help readers find our campgrounds, I've provided GPS coordinates for each entrance. More accurately known as UTM coordinates, the numbers index a specific point using a grid method. The survey datum used to arrive at the coordinates is WGS84. The UTM coordinates provided with the campground profile may be entered directly into a hand-held or car GPS unit; just make sure the unit is set to navigate using the UTM system in conjunction with WGS84 datum. Now you can navigate directly to the entrance. *Note:* The address listed in the key information box directs you to further information and is not necessarily the campground address.

Readers can easily access all campgrounds in this book by using the directions given, the overview map, and the campsite maps, which show at least one major road leading into the area. But for those who enjoy using the latest GPS technology to navigate, the necessary data has been provided. A brief explanation of the UTM coordinates follows.

UTM COORDINATES: ZONE, EASTING, AND NORTHING

In the UTM coordinates box on the first page of each hike are three numbers labeled zone, easting, and northing. Here's an example from Merchants Millpond State Park (page 108):

UTM Zone (WGS84)   18S
Easting   0349570
Northing   4032730

The zone number (18) refers to one of the 60 longitudinal zones (vertical) of a map using the Universal Transverse Mercator (UTM) projection. Each zone is 6 degrees wide. The zone letter (S) refers to one of the 20 latitudinal zones (horizontal) that span from 80° South to 84° North.

The easting number (0349570) references in meters how far east the point is from the zero value for eastings, which runs north-south through Greenwich, England. Increasing easting coordinates on a topographical map or on your GPS screen indicate that you are moving east; decreasing easting coordinates indicate that you are moving west.

In the northern hemisphere, the northing number (4032730) references in meters how far you are from the equator. On a topo map or GPS receiver, increasing northing numbers indicate you are traveling north.

In the southern hemisphere, the northing number references how far you are from a latitude line that is 10 million meters south of the equator. On a topo map or GPS receiver, decreasing northing coordinates indicate you are traveling south.

FIRST-AID KIT

A useful first-aid kit may contain more items than you might think necessary. These are just the basics. Prepackaged kits in waterproof bags (Atwater Carey and Adventure Medical make them) are available. As a preventive measure, take along sunscreen and insect repellent. Even though quite a few items are listed here, they pack down into a small space:

Ace bandages or Spenco joint wraps	Butterfly-closure bandages
Adhesive bandages, such as Band-Aids	Comb and tweezers (for removing ticks from your skin)
Antibiotic ointment (Neosporin or the generic equivalent)	Emergency poncho
Antiseptic or disinfectant, such as Betadine or hydrogen peroxide	Epinephrine in a prefilled syringe (for people known to have severe allergic reactions to such things as bee stings)
Aspirin or acetaminophen	Gauze (one roll)
Benadryl or the generic equivalent, diphenhydramine (in case of allergic reactions)	Gauze compress pads (six 4- x 4-inch pads)

SNAKES

North Carolina is home to 37 varieties of snakes, 6 of which are poisonous: the coral snake, cottonmouth, copperhead, diamondback rattler, pygmy rattler, timber rattler, scarlet

RATTLESNAKE

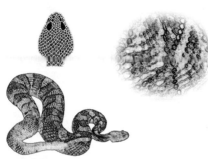

COPPERHEAD

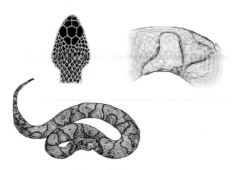

snake, and scarlet Kingsnake. South Carolina has three poisonous snakes among its varieties: the timber rattler, copperhead, and Eastern diamondback rattler. The first two are found throughout the state, while the last one is found in the coastal plain. A good rule of thumb is to give whatever animal you encounter a wide berth and leave it alone.

TICKS

Ticks like to hang out in the brush that grows along trails. They are common in the woodlands of the Piedmont of North Carolina and Midlands of South Carolina. You should be tick-aware during the warm season. Ticks, actually arthropods and not insects, are ectoparasites, which need a host for the majority of their life cycle in order to reproduce. The ticks that light onto you while hiking will be very small, sometimes so tiny that you won't be able to spot them. Primarily of two varieties, deer ticks and dog ticks, both need a few hours of actual attachment before they can transmit any disease they may harbor. I've found ticks in my socks and on my legs several hours after a hike that have not yet anchored. If you've been in tick country, the best strategy is to visually check every half hour or so while hiking, do a thorough check before you get in the car, and then, when you take a post-hike shower, do an even more thorough check of your entire body. Ticks that haven't latched on are easily removed but not easily killed. If I pick off a tick in the woods, I just toss it aside. If I find one on my person at home, I dispatch it and then send it down the toilet. For ticks that have embedded, removal with tweezers is best.

POISONOUS PLANTS

Recognizing poison ivy, oak, and sumac and avoiding contact with them are the most effective ways to prevent the painful, itchy rashes associated with these plants. In the Southeast, poison ivy ranges from a thick, tree-hugging vine to a shaded groundcover, three leaflets to a leaf; poison oak occurs as either a vine or shrub, with three leaflets as well; and poison sumac flourishes in swampland, each leaf containing 7 to 13 leaflets. Urushiol, the oil in the sap of these plants, is responsible for the rash. Usually within 12 to 14 hours of exposure (but sometimes much later), raised lines and/or blisters will appear, accompanied by a terrible itch. Refrain from scratching because bacteria under fingernails can cause infection. Wash and dry the rash thoroughly, applying a calamine lotion or other product to help dry out the rash. If itching or blistering is severe, seek medical attention. Remember that oil-contaminated clothes, pets, or hiking gear can easily cause an irritating rash on you or someone else, so wash not only any exposed parts of your body but also clothes, gear, and pets.

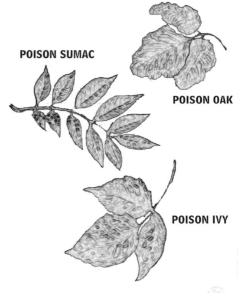

POISON SUMAC

POISON OAK

POISON IVY

MOSQUITOES

Mosquitoes are common in the Carolinas, mountainous regions of both states excepted. Skeeters along with no-see-ums can plague coastal areas. Although it's very rare, individuals can become infected with the West Nile virus by being bitten by an infected mosquito. Culex mosquitoes, the primary varieties that can transmit West Nile virus to humans, thrive in urban rather than natural areas. They lay their eggs in stagnant water and can breed in any standing water that remains for more than five days. Most people infected with West Nile virus have no symptoms of illness, but some may become ill, usually 3 to 15 days after being bitten.

Anytime you expect mosquitoes to be buzzing around, you may want to wear protective clothing, such as long sleeves, long pants, and socks. Loose-fitting, light-colored clothing is best. Spray clothing with insect repellent. Remember to follow the instructions on the repellent and to take extra care with children.

HELPFUL HINTS

To make the most of your tent-camping trip, call ahead whenever possible. If going to a state or national park, call for an informative brochure before setting out. This way you can familiarize yourself with the area. Once there, ask questions. Most stewards of the land are proud of their terra firma and are happy to help you have the best time possible.

If traveling in the national forests of the Carolinas, call ahead and order a forest map. Not only will a map make it that much easier to reach your destination, but nearby hikes, scenic drives, waterfalls, and landmarks will also be easier to find. There are forest visitor centers in addition to ranger stations. Call or visit and ask questions. When ordering a map, ask for any additional literature about the area in which you are interested.

In writing this book, I had the pleasure of meeting many friendly, helpful people: local residents proud of the unique lands around them, and state park and national forest employees who endured my endless questions. Even better were my fellow tent campers, who were eager to share their knowledge about their favorite spots. They already know what beauty lies on the horizon.

As the Carolinas become more populated, these lands become that much more precious. Enjoy them, protect them, and use them wisely.

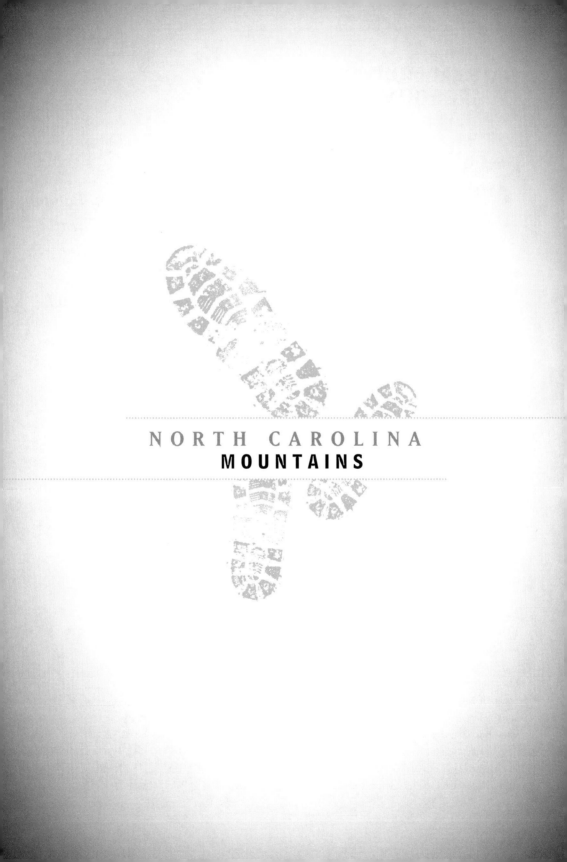

NORTH CAROLINA
MOUNTAINS

BALSAM MOUNTAIN CAMPGROUND

THE RARE SPRUCE-FIR FOREST that cloaks the highest elevations of the Smoky Mountains are among the primary reasons this mountain range was designated a national park. Covering 13,000 of the park's 500,000 acres, the forest composes the southern limit of this relic of the Ice Age. More than 10,000 years ago, when glaciers covered much of the United States, woodlands much more reminiscent of those in Canada today migrated south. When the glaciers retreated, this forest survived on the highest points of the Smokies, creating an "island" of red spruce and Fraser fir trees.

So what does this have to do with tent camping? Well, it just so happens that Balsam Mountain Campground is located in a swath of this rare forest. Not only does it offer the highest tent camping within Great Smoky Mountains National Park, but it also offers campers a chance to experience this remarkable forest firsthand.

The campground was set up not long after the inception of the national park in 1934. Back then, few visitors drove or pulled oversize campers on the narrow, winding roads; the majority tent camped. So when the campground was set up, builders had tent campers in mind. Today, we can camp in the fine tradition of the first park visitors.

Laid out in a classic loop, Balsam Mountain sits on a rib ridge between the headwaters of Flat and Bunches creeks. Past the entrance station, campsites are set along the main road.

You will immediately notice the sites' small size, a historic element of Balsam Mountain that discourages most of today's RV campers. But even with the small sites relatively close together, you will find ample privacy because the campground rarely fills.

Keeping south on the main road, come to a loop. Campsites are spread along this loop among the fir and spruce trees. The ground slopes off steeply away

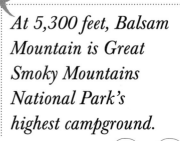

At 5,300 feet, Balsam Mountain is Great Smoky Mountains National Park's highest campground.

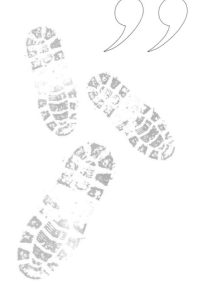

RATINGS

Beauty: ✩ ✩ ✩ ✩
Privacy: ✩ ✩ ✩
Spaciousness: ✩ ✩
Quiet: ✩ ✩ ✩ ✩
Security: ✩ ✩ ✩ ✩
Cleanliness: ✩ ✩ ✩ ✩

ADDRESS:	107 Park HQ Rd. Gatlinburg, TN 37738
OPERATED BY:	National Park Service
INFORMATION:	(865) 436-1200; nps.gov/grsm
OPEN:	Mid-May–late September
SITES:	45
EACH SITE:	Picnic table, fire grate
ASSIGNMENT:	First come, first served; no reservations
REGISTRATION:	Self-registration
FACILITIES:	Water spigot, flush toilet
PARKING:	At campsites only
FEE:	$14
ELEVATION:	5,300 feet
RESTRICTIONS:	*Pets:* On leash only *Fires:* In fire grates only *Alcohol:* At campsite only *Vehicles:* 30-foot trailer-length limit *Other:* 7-day stay limit

from the road, resulting in some unlevel sites. With a little scouting, however, you will find a good site among the evergreens.

Balsam Mountain is off the beaten national park path. In fact, the road leading to the campground connects to the Blue Ridge Parkway, which then connects to the main body of the park. There is only one trail in the area, but it is a winner: Flat Creek. Leave the Heintooga Picnic Area on this path, and enjoy a magnificent view of the main Smokies crest before descending to the perched watershed of Flat Creek. Cruise through an attractive high-elevation forest before reaching the side trail to Flat Creek Falls, a steep and narrow cascade. Backtrack or continue past the falls to cross Bunches Creek and reach Balsam Mountain Road.

Balsam Mountain Road, just one of many interesting forest drives in the immediate area, leads 8 miles to the Blue Ridge Parkway, the granddaddy of all scenic roads in the Southern Appalachian Mountains, with recreation opportunities to both the north and south. A more rustic forest drive leaves Heintooga Picnic Area on a gravel road and runs north along Balsam Mountain before descending into Straight Fork valley to emerge at the nearby Qualla Cherokee Indian Reservation. Several hiking trails are along the way, including Palmer Creek Trail—which descends into a beautiful, richly forested valley—and Hyatt Ridge Trail, which, along with Beech Gap Trail, makes for a rewarding high-country loop hike of 8 miles. Anglers can fish for trout on Straight Fork or enjoy many of the stream- and pond-fishing opportunities on the reservation. The nearby town of Cherokee has your typical Smokies tourist traps as well as camping supplies.

MAP

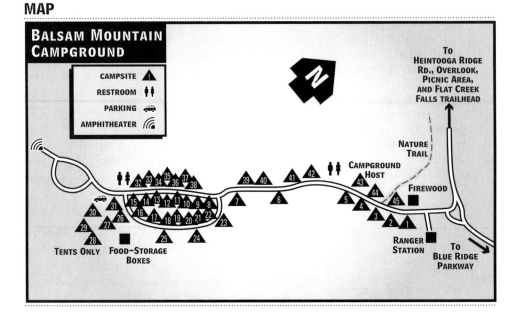

BALSAM MOUNTAIN CAMPGROUND

CAMPSITE

RESTROOM

PARKING

AMPHITHEATER

To HEINTOOGA RIDGE RD., OVERLOOK, PICNIC AREA, AND FLAT CREEK FALLS TRAILHEAD

NATURE TRAIL

CAMPGROUND HOST

FIREWOOD

TENTS ONLY

FOOD-STORAGE BOXES

RANGER STATION

To BLUE RIDGE PARKWAY

GETTING THERE

From the Oconaluftee Visitor Center near Cherokee, take Newfound Gap Road 0.5 miles south to the Blue Ridge Parkway. Turn left onto the Blue Ridge Parkway, and follow it 10.8 miles to Heintooga Ridge Road. Turn left on Heintooga Ridge Road, and drive 8 miles to Balsam Mountain Campground, on your left.

GPS COORDINATES

UTM Zone (WGS84) 17S

Easting 0301570

Northing 3933370

Latitude 35 33' 54.1"

Longitude 83 10' 27.9"

2
BIG CREEK CAMPGROUND

Only tents are allowed at this walk-in campground located in the Smokies' remote Far East.

GREAT SMOKY MOUNTAINS NATIONAL PARK has a reputation, somewhat undeserved, of being overcrowded. Sure, some places can seem a bit peopled, but if you know the right places to go, your time in the park can be a relaxing getaway. Big Creek Campground is one of those places. It is the Smokies' smallest campground and its sole tent-only campground. This walk-in campground is set deep in the woods adjacent to the pure mountain waters of Big Creek—so deep, in fact, that when you come to the campground parking area, you'll wonder where the campground is. (For your information, it's between the campground parking area and noisy Big Creek.)

A small footpath leaves the parking area and loops the 12 campsites in the shade of tall hardwoods. Since Big Creek is a walk-in campground, you must tote your camping supplies anywhere from 100 to 300 feet. But after that, you'll be hearing only the intonations of Big Creek and smelling the wildflowers rather than hearing RV engines and smelling exhaust fumes.

Five of the sites are directly creekside. Each is spacious enough for you to spread out your gear. The new tent pads are elevated and well drained. A somewhat-sparse understory reduces privacy, but the intimate walk-in setup magnifies an atmosphere of camaraderie among fellow campers not necessarily found in larger drive-in campgrounds.

The campground comfort station borders the parking area. It houses flush toilets and a large sink with a cold-water faucet. Two other water spigots are found along the footpath loop. A recycling bin is located in the parking area. A pay phone is located 1 mile back down the gravel road at the Big Creek Ranger Station. You can acquire limited supplies a bit farther down Big Creek at Mountain Momma's Country Store, but try to bring in what you need; this way, you can spend your time enjoying the park.

RATINGS

Beauty: ☆ ☆ ☆ ☆ ☆
Privacy: ☆ ☆ ☆
Spaciousness: ☆ ☆ ☆ ☆
Quiet: ☆ ☆ ☆ ☆ ☆
Security: ☆ ☆ ☆ ☆
Cleanliness: ☆ ☆ ☆ ☆

The Big Creek Trail starts at the campground and traces an old railroad grade from the logging era. Cool off the old-fashioned way in one of the many swimming holes that pool between the white rapids of Big Creek. Gaze up the sides of the valley; the rock bluffs you see have sheltered Smoky Mountain wayfarers for thousands of years. Hike 3.3 miles up Big Creek to find the tumbling cascades of Mouse Creek Falls. Falls often occur where a feeder creek enters a main stream; the primary stream valley erodes faster than the side stream valley, creating a hanging side canyon and then a waterfall. Continue on to Walnut Bottoms at 5 miles. This area has historically had more man-bear encounters than anywhere in the park, so keep all food locked in your trunk, not in the seat of your car, when away from camp. Crestmont Logging Company had a camp here in the early 1900s, but now the area has returned to its former splendor. If you wish to explore further, three other trails splinter from Walnut Bottoms.

How about a strenuous hike through old-growth forest to a mountaintop capped by a Canadian-type forest with a 360-degree view from a fire tower? It's 6 miles up the Baxter Creek Trail, but your efforts will be amply rewarded. Start at the Big Creek picnic area just below the campground and go for it. Or take Mount Sterling Trail from Mount Sterling Gap on nearby NC 284. It's only 3 miles to the tower this way. Just up from the Big Creek Ranger Station is Chestnut Branch Trail. It leads 2 miles to the highest and wildest section of the entire Appalachian Trail, which traverses the Smoky Mountains. The historic fire tower at Mount Cammerer is only 4 miles farther. Or loop back on the Appalachian Trail to Davenport Gap, and road-walk a short piece back to the campground.

Big Creek is wilderness tent camping at its best. The walk-in setting is your first step into the natural world of the Smokies. The rest of your adventure is limited only by your desire to explore the 500,000 acres in Big Creek Campground's backyard.

KEY INFORMATION

ADDRESS:	107 Park HQ Rd. Gatlinburg, TN 37738
OPERATED BY:	Great Smoky Mountains National Park
INFORMATION:	(865) 436-1200; nps.gov/gsrm
OPEN:	Mid-March–October
SITES:	12
EACH SITE:	Picnic table, fire pit, lantern post
ASSIGNMENT:	First come, first served; no reservations
REGISTRATION:	Self-registration
FACILITIES:	Cold water flush toilets
PARKING:	At individual sites
FEE:	$14
ELEVATION:	1,700 feet
RESTRICTIONS:	*Pets:* On leash only *Fires:* In fire pits only *Alcohol:* At campsite only *Vehicles:* No RVs or trailers *Other:* 7-day stay limit

MAP

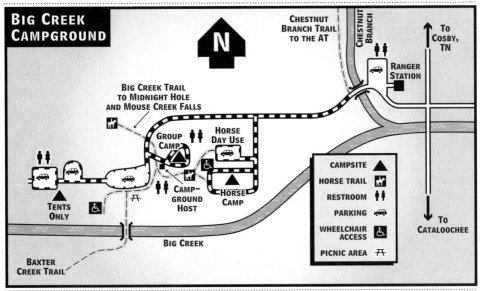

GETTING THERE

From Cove Creek in Tennessee, take I-40 west 15 miles, crossing the state line, to Exit 451/Waterville. Cross the Pigeon River and turn left to follow the Pigeon upstream. Come to an intersection 2.3 miles after crossing the Pigeon. Proceed forward through the intersection and soon enter the park. Pass the Big Creek Ranger Station, and drive to the end of the gravel road and the campground after 3.5 miles.

GPS COORDINATES

UTM Zone (WGS84) 17S

Easting 0309210

Northing 3958210

Latitude 35 45' 5.6"

Longitude 83 6' 35.3"

3
CABLE COVE CAMPGROUND

RECENT HISTORY IS A THEME of sorts for this charming and sedate campground, which sits on former farmland once tilled by the Cable family. After World War II began, the demand for aluminum and the power to manufacture it soared, leading to the construction of nearby Fontana Dam. Begun in 1942 and used to generate power to produce aluminum for the war, the dam remains an important source of energy. Prior to flooding behind the dam, the farming families moved away. The U.S. Forest Service moved in, later establishing a campground in the hollow.

Cable Cove's proximity to Fontana Lake makes it an ideal camp from which to visit the Smoky Mountains via boat, thus avoiding auto traffic. Fontana is a lightly used lake, with unlimited views of the park that are unspoiled by the troops of tourists that fill the highways on busy summer weekends.

Cable Cove Campground stretches out along a gravel road that slopes down toward Fontana Lake, a half mile away. A small loop at the end of the campground road enables drivers to turn around; this loop holds five campsites. Cable Creek, a small trout stream, parallels the road on the right. The campground is well maintained, quiet, and unassuming. Shortly after arriving, I felt as if I belonged there, like one of the neighbors.

The 10 creekside sites are heavily wooded and have a thick understory. They are spacious yet have an air of privacy because of the junglelike vegetation along Cable Creek. The 11 sites opposite the creek have a grassy, gladelike understory beneath second-growth trees that are reclaiming the old fields. During my stay, the grass had been freshly trimmed and looked especially attractive. This "yard" space makes for a more open camping area, one conducive to visiting your neighbor, a customary thing to do in friendly

> *Stay at Cable Cove and access the Smoky Mountains National Park by boat or land, free of traffic hassles.*

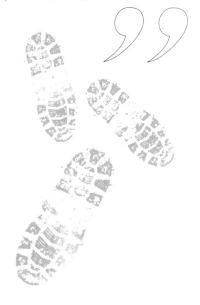

RATINGS

Beauty: ✪ ✪ ✪ ✪
Privacy: ✪ ✪ ✪
Spaciousness: ✪ ✪ ✪ ✪ ✪
Quiet: ✪ ✪ ✪ ✪
Security: ✪ ✪ ✪ ✪
Cleanliness: ✪ ✪ ✪ ✪

ADDRESS: Cheoah Ranger District
1133 Massey Branch Rd.
Robbinsville, NC 28771

OPERATED BY: U.S. Forest Service

INFORMATION: (704) 479-6431; cs.unca.edu/nfsnc

OPEN: April 14– October 31

SITES: 26

EACH SITE: Tent pad, lantern post, picnic table, fire grate

ASSIGNMENT: First come, first served; no reservations

REGISTRATION: Self-registration on site

FACILITIES: Water, low-volume flush toilet

PARKING: At campsites only

FEE: $10

ELEVATION: 1,800 feet

RESTRICTIONS: *Pets:* On leash only
Fires: In fire grates only
Alcohol: At campsites only
Vehicles: None
Other: 14-day stay limit

western North Carolina. These campsites are some of the largest I have ever seen, extending far back from the road. An area of brush and trees divides the upper and lower campgrounds. Beyond the brush are the five sites at the turn-around loop, in the deep woods adjacent to Cable Creek.

Three water spigots have been placed at even intervals in the linear campground. Two comfort stations with flush toilets are at either end of the campground; campers in the middle may have to walk a bit to use them. But even this stroll could be an opportunity to get to know your neighbor. I camped toward the middle, and by the time I left, the gravel road resembled a country lane—slow moving and full of good friends.

Most of them will be boaters. A high-quality boat ramp is a half mile away; campers use it to fish for bream, bass, trout, and walleye, as well as to access the national park. (Using a boat to access the park is a smart way to beat the crowds. I've been doing it for two decades and wonder why it hasn't caught on more.) Several hiking trails in the Smokies run right down to the lake. Check out the 360-degree view from Shuckstack Fire Tower. To reach the tower, which is visible from the lake, boat up the Eagle Creek arm of Fontana Lake. From the embayment, the Lost Cove Trail leads 3 miles up to the Appalachian Trail. Just 0.4 miles south on the Appalachian Trail is the tower. The outline of Fontana Lake is easily discerned from the tower. Look northeast and see the spine of the Smokies until it fades from view.

Across the water from Cable Cove is famed Hazel Creek, whose trout waters have been featured in fishing magazines for years. But don't visit just for the fish. Hike up the gentle trail that parallels the creek to discover relics of the Smokies' past, including old homesites, fields, and mining endeavors. Wide bridges spanning the creek make this walk even more pleasant. You can only access this end of the Appalachian Trail by boat; if you don't have one, contact Fontana Marina at (704) 498-2211, extension 277, to arrange for a shuttle. The marina is only 4 miles west of Cable Cove. You can purchase limited supplies at the small store at Fontana Village Resort near the marina, but you're better off

MAP

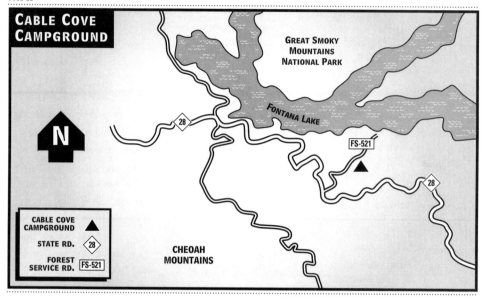

CABLE COVE
CAMPGROUND

GREAT SMOKY
MOUNTAINS
NATIONAL PARK

N

28

FONTANA LAKE

FS-521

28

CABLE COVE
CAMPGROUND ▲

STATE RD. ◇28◇

FOREST
SERVICE RD. FS-521

CHEOAH
MOUNTAINS

stocking up in Maryville, Tennessee, if you are coming from the Volunteer State, or in Robbinsville, North Carolina, south of Cable Cove on NC 143.

Also near the marina is the engineering marvel that is Fontana Dam, the tallest dam east of the Rockies at 480 feet, and well worth a visit. A visitor center recounts the story of the dam, and cable cars take visitors down to its powerhouse. You can cross the dam in your auto—the landlubber's way to access the Smokies—at one of the more remote trailheads. Trace the Appalachian Trail 3.3 miles up to Shuckstack and its tower. Or take the undulating Lakeshore Trail through the Smokies' lush flora 5 miles to Eagle Creek and its embayment. Whether you get there by land or water, this slice of the Smokies is a gem to visit.

GETTING THERE

From Fontana Village take NC 28 east 4.7 miles. Turn left on FS 521 1.5 miles. Cable Cove will be on your right.

GPS COORDINATES

UTM Zone (WGS84) 17S
Easting 0250160
Northing 3924300
Latitude 35 24' 41.1"
Longitude 83 46' 28.3"

4
CATALOOCHEE CAMPGROUND

> *Cataloochee Valley's remoteness and inaccessibility make it one of the Smokies' better-kept secrets.*

CATALOOCHEE CAMPGROUND is only the first attractive spot you'll see in this valley of meadows, streams, mountains, history—and elk, which have been introduced into the valley and offer extraordinary wildlife viewing in Cataloochee's meadows. The celebrated fishing waters of Cataloochee Creek form one border of the campground, while a small feeder stream forms the other. In between is a flat, attractive camping area canopied with stately white pines.

The campground has ideal summer weather, with warm days and cool nights. An elevation of 2,600 feet is fairly high for a valley campground with a stream the size of Cataloochee Creek. Cataloochee uses the basic campground design: campsites splintering off a loop road. Six of the sites lie along Cataloochee Creek; a few others border the small feeder stream. All are roomy and placed where the pines allow. An erratic understory of hemlock and rhododendron leaves privacy to the luck of which site you draw. The campground host is situated at the entrance for your safety and convenience. Be forewarned: Bears are sighted yearly at this campground, so properly store your food and keep the wild in the Smoky Mountain bears.

Most RV campers shy away from this campground because the National Park Service advises against RVs making the long drive over rough, gravel roads. Cataloochee fills up on summer weekends, yet with only 27 sites, it doesn't seem overly crowded. A comfort station is next to the campground at the head of the host. It has flush toilets and a cold-water faucet that pours into a large sink. Another water spigot is at the other end of the campground.

With all there is to do, you'll probably stay here only to rest from perusing the park. The first order of business is an auto tour of Cataloochee Valley. To gain

RATINGS

Beauty: ✪ ✪ ✪ ✪ ✪
Privacy: ✪ ✪ ✪ ✪
Spaciousness: ✪ ✪ ✪ ✪ ✪
Quiet: ✪ ✪ ✪ ✪ ✪
Security: ✪ ✪ ✪ ✪
Cleanliness: ✪ ✪ ✪ ✪

a feel for the area, get a copy of the handy park-service pamphlet at the Ranger Station. An old church, a school, and numerous homesites are a delight to explore. Informative displays further explain about life long ago in this part of the world.

Cataloochee Valley is a hiker's paradise. Take the Boogerman Trail 7.4 undulating miles through different vegetation zones. The trail, which begins and ends at Caldwell Fork Trail, loops among old-growth hemlocks and tulip trees. Old homesites add a touch of human history; numerous footbridges make exploring this watery mountain land fun and easy on the feet. Or take the Little Cataloochee Trail to Little Cataloochee Church. Set in the backwoods, the church was built in 1890 and is still used today. Other signs of humanity that you'll see include a ramshackle cabin, chimneys, fence posts, and rock walls.

The Cataloochee Divide Trail starts at 4,000 feet and rambles along the ridgeline border that straddles the Maggie and Cataloochee valleys. To the north is the rugged green expanse of the national park, and to the south are the developed areas along US 19. Grassy knolls along the way make good viewing and relaxing spots.

Using the Rough Fork, Caldwell Fork, and Fork Ridge trails, you can make another loop, this one 9.3 miles. Pass the fields of the Woody Place; then climb Fork Ridge, descend to Caldwell Fork, and climb Fork Ridge yet again to experience the literal highs and lows of Appalachian hiking.

The meadows of Cataloochee Valley are an ideal setting for a picnic. Decide on your favorite view and lay down your blanket. Nearby shady streams will serenade you as you look up at the wooded ridges that line the valley. Elk, deer, and other critters feed at the edges of the fields, drawing in nature photographers. Dusk is an ideal time to see Cataloochee's wildlife.

During our last stay at this campground, summer weather had finally hit. The air had a lazy, hazy feel as we toured the valley's historic structures. I fished away the afternoon, catching and releasing a few rainbows downstream from the campground. After grilling hamburgers for supper, we walked up Rough Fork Trail to the Woody Place. The homestead looked picturesque

KEY INFORMATION

ADDRESS:	107 Park HQ Rd. Gatlinburg, TN 37738
OPERATED BY:	Great Smoky Mountains National Park
INFORMATION:	(865) 436-1200; nps.gov/grsm
OPEN:	Mid-March–October
SITES:	27
EACH SITE:	Picnic table, fire pit, lantern post
ASSIGNMENT:	First come, first served; no reservations
REGISTRATION:	Self-registration on site
FACILITIES:	Cold water, flush toilets
PARKING:	At individual sites
FEE:	$17
ELEVATION:	2,610 feet
RESTRICTIONS:	*Pets:* On leash only *Fires:* In fire pits only *Alcohol:* At campsites only *Vehicles:* None *Other:* 7-day stay limit

MAP

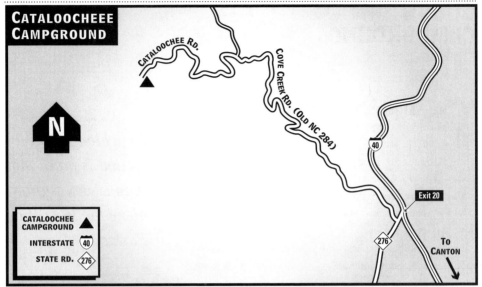

CATALOOCHEEE CAMPGROUND

CATALOOCHEE RD.

COVE CREEK RD. (OLD NC 284)

40

Exit 20

276

To CANTON

N

CATALOOCHEE CAMPGROUND	▲
INTERSTATE	40
STATE RD.	276

GETTING THERE

From Canton, drive 11 miles west on I-40 to Exit 20; then drive west on NC 276. Follow it a short distance, then turn right on Cove Creek Road, which you follow nearly 6 miles to enter the park. Two miles beyond the park boundary, turn left onto the paved Cataloochee Road, and follow it 3 miles. The campground will be on your left.

as the late-evening sunlight filtered through the nearby forest. As we came back to the trailhead, deer browsed in the Cataloochee meadow. We knew we had come to the right place. So will you.

GPS COORDINATES

UTM Zone (WGS84) 17S

Easting 0312066

Northing 3946361

Latitude 35 38' 42.5"

Longitude 83 4' 32.7"

5
DOUGHTON CAMPGROUND

THE NATIONAL PARK SERVICE does a really good job with this Blue Ridge Parkway campground, which is located on the crest of the Blue Ridge and has a mountaintop ambience. A smart design spreads out over 100-plus sites and makes the area seem like several small campgrounds. Dividing the tent and RV sites into separate sections makes it even better.

The 6,430-acre park and campground are named after former North Carolina Rep. "Muley Bob" Doughton, who fought hard to help the parkway become the scenic reality it is. He would be proud of this area, which unobtrusively integrates modern structures into the historic dwellings and hiking trails that lace the park.

Before you explore Doughton Park, pick a campsite. This may take a few minutes, as the campground has six distinct areas. Open and airy, it is tastefully landscaped and well integrated into the ridgetop setting. Even the most discriminating tent campers will find a site to suit their tastes.

The first loop holds 22 sites and is heavily wooded, yet with a light understory. The sites undulate along a hill and are fairly close, so you may be a tad cozy with your neighbor. The comfort station is a ways down a sloping path, possibly a little farther than some are willing to walk.

Sites 23 through 33 are set back in the woods, down from the paved campground road. Short paths lead back to them, so you will have to carry your gear to your site. This distance allows for the most rustic camping experience, out of sight from vehicles. The sites closest to the parking area border a grassy field adjacent to the parking area. Campers share the comfort station with the first loop via a short, paved path.

The second loop circles the highest point of the campground. It has 30 sites and is centered on a grassy

> *Doughton Campground is much more than a way station along the Blue Ridge Parkway.*

RATINGS

Beauty: ✰ ✰ ✰ ✰
Privacy: ✰ ✰ ✰
Spaciousness: ✰ ✰ ✰
Quiet: ✰ ✰ ✰
Security: ✰ ✰ ✰ ✰
Cleanliness: ✰ ✰ ✰ ✰ ✰

KEY INFORMATION

ADDRESS: 199 Hemphill Knob Rd. Asheville, NC 28801

OPERATED BY: National Park Service

INFORMATION: (828) 298-0398; nps.gov/blri

OPEN: Mid-May–October

SITES: 135 tent and RV sites

EACH SITE: Tent pad, fire ring, picnic table

ASSIGNMENT: First come, first served; no reservations

REGISTRATION: At campground hut

FACILITIES: Water, flush toilets, pay phone

PARKING: At campsites only

FEE: $16

ELEVATION: 3,600 feet

RESTRICTIONS: *Pets:* On 6-foot or shorter leash
Fires: In fire rings only
Alcohol: At campsites only
Vehicles: None
Other: 14-day stay limit, 30-day total limit for calendar year

glade where a water tank sits. Oddly enough, a campsite is located right by the water tank; when I checked it out, I found the view of the surrounding mountain lands worth the intrusion of the green structure. Other sites here offer intermittent views of the Blue Ridge and beyond. You even have a view from the comfort station at the loop's center.

The main loop continues along the ridge and passes a few sites for larger pop-up tent campers, then enters the campfire circle loop. Its nine sites are situated in an attractive meadow. Trees have been strategically planted by each campsite for shade and aesthetic appeal.

Beyond the campfire circle loop is yet another loop that winds amid hilly forestland, rolling and dipping among rock outcrops. There are 20 sites here, situated where the land allows. Because the loop is at the very back of the campground, you will encounter few vehicles casually driving by to their respective sites. A comfort station is centered on this loop as well.

Back on the main loop, in an open area backed against woodland, are 11 more sites for larger pop-ups. For such a large campground, there is a curious lack of faucets—there are only six, and they could have been better placed. But this is a minor inconvenience for this well-kept, secure campground that is 90 percent tent campers. A campground host lives on-site.

The Blue Ridge Parkway is an exercise in scenic beauty, but I think this particular area is exceptional even for the BRP. A drive in either direction will sate your taste for dramatic landscapes and historic sites. The Brinegar Cabin is just a short distance north. Of course, the most rewarding views are those earned with a little sweat.

Doughton Park has more than 30 miles of trails that meander through pastures, along wooded ridges, and by mountain streams. The Bluff Mountain Trail departs from the campground and gives you a sampling of this country. It extends for 3 or so miles in each direction. The Fodderstack Trail, a 2-mile round trip, climbs to the Wildcat Rocks Overlook. Another recommended trail is Basin Creek, which ends at the Caudill Cabin (only accessible by foot). Cedar Ridge Trail begins at the Brinegar Cabin and drops down to Basin

MAP

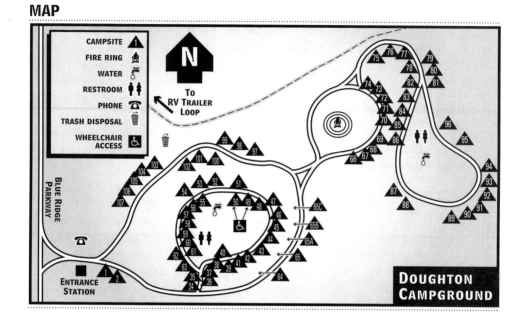

Creek. Before you hike any of these trails, though, stop at the campground hut and pick up a free trail map. Get out there and stretch your legs after enjoying that fantastic Blue Ridge Parkway scenery.

GETTING THERE

Take NC 18 west from Sparta 14 miles to the Blue Ridge Parkway. Turn north on the parkway, and drive 6 miles to milepost 239. Doughton Park Campground will be on your left.

GPS COORDINATES

UTM Zone (WGS84) 17S

Easting 0484187

Northing 4031470

Latitude 36 24' 25.9"

Longitude 81 15' 0.1"

> *Hanging Dog sits by picturesque Hiwassee Lake, nestled in the rural mountains of western North Carolina.*

RATINGS

Beauty: ✪ ✪ ✪ ✪
Privacy: ✪ ✪ ✪ ✪
Spaciousness: ✪ ✪ ✪ ✪ ✪
Quiet: ✪ ✪ ✪
Security: ✪ ✪ ✪
Cleanliness: ✪ ✪ ✪ ✪

WHEN PEOPLE THINK OF SMOKY MOUNTAIN country, they picture rolling mountains, deep forests, and rushing streams. That's what comes naturally. However, when early settlers came here, they started the unnatural job of building dams. The hilly terrain of the Southern Appalachians proved to be fertile ground for creating lakes. Later, the Tennessee Valley Authority dammed waters on a grand scale. Now we have an abundance of scenic lakes that seemingly have mountains growing right out of them. Much of the land around these lakes is owned by you and me, courtesy of the U.S. Forest Service. Along some lakes, the Forest Service has built campgrounds that enable us to enjoy some of these bodies of water. Hanging Dog Campground is just such a place.

Hanging Dog was named after a nearby creek of the same name that flows through a parcel of the neighboring Cherokee reservation. Legend has it that a brave dog was accidentally snared in the creek while chasing a deer to provide meat for the hungry people. The dog survived, and the people named the area to commemorate the canine's actions.

The campground features four widely separated loops, each of which is almost like its own campground. A dry pine-oak forest covers the peninsula that borders Hiwassee Lake. Adequate yet sparse, water supplies and comfort stations are placed in every loop.

This Civilian Conservation Corps–era campground has aged well. Vegetation cultivated over many decades provides ideal campground aesthetics, and in this relaxed atmosphere time seems to move slowly. Adults who first visited Hanging Dog as children pass on the joys of camping here to the next generation.

Loop A spurs off to the right of the campground's main road and circles a hollow formed by a tiny stream. The lower reaches of the loop are piney and open. The vegetation thickens farther up the hollow, allowing for more privacy. The campsites here are well established and spacious. Landscaping timbers have been strategically placed to help with site leveling and delineation.

Loop B forms a figure eight along an arm of Hiwassee Lake. The 15 sites here are in a grassy glade beneath tall pines. The five most popular sites in this loop fit snugly against the lake.

Pass over quite a few speed bumps to reach Loop C. It also forms a crude figure eight and is a long walk down the main campground road from the first two loops. Enter an open pine forest with spacious campsites. The back side of the loop runs along a small rhododendron-choked branch that provides a denser understory and increased site privacy.

Loop D is across the road from Loop C in some rolling woods. It offers the most densely forested sites, with a thick understory of mountain laurel and small trees. The loop is now used as a picnic area and for overflow camping when all the other sites are taken, which is a shame because it's the most attractive loop.

Hiwassee Lake's 180 miles of picturesque wooded shoreline are primarily under U.S. Forest Service stewardship, minimizing development. Bass, bream, and crappie are among the species that provide excellent fishing in these mountain lakes. The transparent green waters will lure you in for a swim on a hot summer day. Boaters can access the lake via the boat ramp at the very end of the main campground road.

Two hiking trails meander from the campground around the peninsula. The Mingus Trail starts across from Loop B and runs through pine-oak woods down to the boat ramp, from which you can return to your campsite on the road. The Ramsey Bluff Trail starts at the back of Loop B and winds along the shore of Hiwassee Lake 2.2 miles and ends at the back of Loop D.

More than just a supply run, the nearby town of Murphy is quintessentially quaint. Absorb the ambience, and make sure to visit the Cherokee County Historical Society Museum, where you can see what life was like in the preindustrial era. You'll find that much of the good from that bygone time is still alive in this slice of Americana.

KEY INFORMATION

ADDRESS:	123 Woodland Dr. Murphy, NC 28906
OPERATED BY:	U.S. Forest Service
INFORMATION:	(828) 837-5152; cs.unca.edu/nfsnc
OPEN:	April–October
SITES:	67
EACH SITE:	Tent pad, fire ring, picnic table, lantern post
ASSIGNMENT:	First come, first served; no reservations
REGISTRATION:	Self-registration on site
FACILITIES:	Water, flush toilets
PARKING:	At campsites only
FEE:	$8
ELEVATION:	1,600 feet
RESTRICTIONS:	*Pets:* On 6-foot or shorter leash *Fires:* In fire rings only *Alcohol:* At campsites only *Vehicles:* At campsites only *Other:* 14-day stay limit; after a 7-day absence, one is allowed to return

MAP

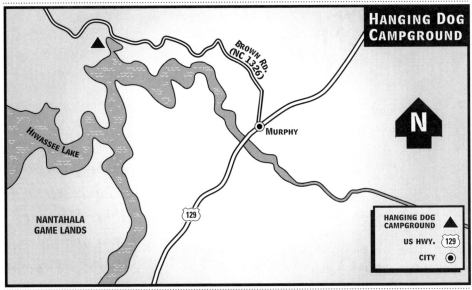

GETTING THERE

From Murphy, take Brown
Road (NC 1326) NW
5 miles. Turn left at campground sign. Hanging Dog
will be straight ahead.

GPS COORDINATES

UTM Zone (WGS84) 16S
Easting 0766130
Northing 3889940
Latitude 35 7' 7.7"
Longitude 84 4' 47.3"

7
HORSE COVE CAMPGROUND

HORSE COVE IS AN UNPRETENTIOUS, small campground adjacent to playful Santeetlah (San-TEE-lah) Creek. Located primarily along Horse Cove Branch, a tributary of Santeetlah Creek, its minimal facilities have an unpolished, old-time feel. In a way, it is two campgrounds: the lower 6 being year-round sites and the upper 11 warm-weather sites. The lower, year-round sites on Santeetlah Creek are across Forest Service Road 416 from the main campground and have a spur road of their own. A pit toilet is the only amenity, although water is available from a spigot in summer and from the creek in winter. These sites overlook Santeetlah Creek from a heavily wooded knoll.

The upper campground runs up a narrow valley carved by Horse Cove Branch, which forms the western campground border. A steep mountainside hems in the campground to the east, but the campsites are graded and kept level with landscaping timbers; this hillside arrangement spreads sites apart both horizontally and vertically. A comfort station with low-flow flush toilets is located at the campground entrance. And you're never far from one of the three water spigots that are conveniently placed about this cozy encampment.

A spare gravel road divides the upper campground. Beneath a hardwood canopy, the five sites beyond Horse Cove Branch are open and dry. They are well spaced along the road, which makes a short loop. The grassy center of the loop has a horseshoe pit. The six sites adjacent to boisterous Horse Cove Branch are isolated from each other by large rocks intermingled with rhododendron and hemlock. The Horse Cove Trail leads to the high country right from the upper campground, then ends and splits into two trails along divergent railroad grades that remain from the logging days.

Stay at Horse Cove Campground and enjoy the lovely trees of Joyce Kilmer Memorial Forest and the Slickrock Wilderness.

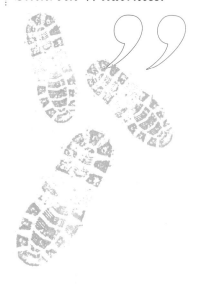

RATINGS

Beauty: ✰ ✰ ✰ ✰
Privacy: ✰ ✰ ✰ ✰
Spaciousness: ✰ ✰ ✰ ✰ ✰
Quiet: ✰ ✰ ✰ ✰
Security: ✰ ✰ ✰
Cleanliness: ✰ ✰ ✰

KEY INFORMATION

ADDRESS:	Cheoah Ranger District 1133 Massey Branch Rd. Robbinsville, NC 28771
OPERATED BY:	U.S. Forest Service
INFORMATION:	(828) 479-6431; cs.unca.edu/nfsnc
OPEN:	Upper campground, April 15–October 31; lower campground, year-round
SITES:	26
EACH SITE:	Tent pad, fire grate, picnic table, lantern post
ASSIGNMENT:	First come, first served; no reservations
REGISTRATION:	Self-registration on site
FACILITIES:	Water in summer only, flush toilets in summer, vault toilets in winter
PARKING:	At individual sites
FEE:	$10 April–October; $5 in winter
ELEVATION:	2,300 feet
RESTRICTIONS:	*Pets:* On leash only *Fires:* In fire grates only *Alcohol:* At campsites only *Vehicles:* None *Other:* 14-day stay limit

The reason for the campground's existence is its proximity to the magnificent Joyce Kilmer Memorial Forest and the adjoining Slickrock Wilderness. Hikers love to walk among the giants of this forest, named for the late writer Joyce Kilmer, who met an untimely end in France during World War I on July 30, 1918. Kilmer is best known for his poem "Trees," the first two lines of which are, "I think that I shall never see / A poem as lovely as a tree."

After Kilmer's death, a nationwide search ensued to locate a forest grand enough to memorialize him. Finally, a tract in North Carolina was selected. What we see today is a 3,800-acre, old-growth woodland that is one of the most impressive remnants of the Southern Appalachians before loggers permanently altered the landscape.

Several trails start at the Joyce Kilmer Memorial Forest parking area, which is 0.7 miles west of the Horse Cove Campground on FS 416. The Joyce Kilmer National Recreation Trail forms a figure eight as it loops through the forest. The 0.8-mile upper loop that travels through Poplar Cove is said to have the densest concentration of large trees in eastern North America. Tulip trees, 20 feet around the base, rise to meet the sun alongside their fellow forest dwellers: hemlock, beech, and oak. The largest cucumber tree in North Carolina is marked with a plaque.

You can't go wrong with any of the three trails that lead out of Joyce Kilmer Memorial Forest into the high country of the Joyce Kilmer–Slickrock Wilderness. A loop hike of differing combinations is possible using any of the Stratton Bald, Naked Ground, and Jenkins Meadow–Hangover Lead trails. For a scenic blockbuster of a hike, take the old Cherokee trading path, known to modern hikers as the Naked Ground Trail. It climbs 4.3 miles to Naked Ground, a spot named for its historical lack of trees. To your left it is 1.3 miles to Bob Stratton Bald, a mile-high mountain meadow with rewarding views of the Smoky and Nantahala forests. When cattle grazing ceased here, the field began to reforest. Later, trees were cut back and native grasses were planted. Consequently, the meadow and its beautiful views were restored. It's my favorite place in this wilderness.

From Naked Ground it is 1.4 miles (right) to

MAP

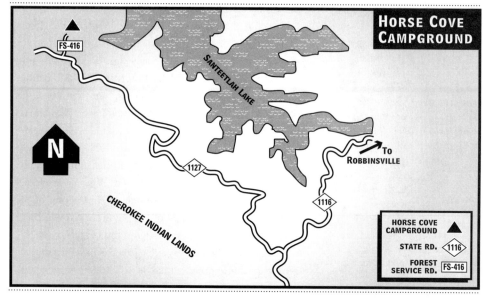

HORSE COVE CAMPGROUND

FS-416

SANTEETLAH LAKE

N

To ROBBINSVILLE

1127

CHEROKEE INDIAN LANDS

1116

HORSE COVE CAMPGROUND

STATE RD. 1116

FOREST SERVICE RD. FS-416

Hangover Lead. This sheer, rocky drop-off needs no assistance from the Forest Service to maintain its views. The Smoky Mountains and Gregory Bald's open field are visible to your right. The lakes and mountains that are the legacy of western North Carolina and eastern Tennessee are all around you. Return via the Naked Ground or Hangover Lead trails.

GETTING THERE

From Robbinsville take US 129 north 1 mile, then turn left on NC 143. Go 3.5 miles to NC 1127, and turn right. Go 12 miles to FS 416, and turn right; FS 416 soon bisects the campground.

GPS COORDINATES

UTM Zone (WGS84) 17S

Easting 0234710

Northing 3917165

Latitude 35 21' 51.3"

Longitude 83 55' 11.0"

8
LAKE JAMES STATE PARK

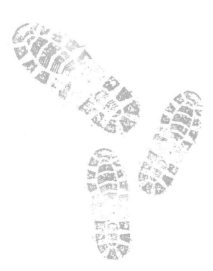

> *All the sites here are walk-ins, and most are directly on Lake James.*

LAKE JAMES, fed by the fine waters of the Pisgah River, is one of the cleanest, clearest lakes in the Carolinas. It also has some of the best views, as the high mountains of the Pisgah National Forest burst skyward beyond the water to the northwest. The contemporary facilities reflect Lake James State Park's status as one of North Carolina's newer public preserves.

The sign for the park on I-40 says, "No RV Camping." I knew then it was a likely inclusion for this book. It's a good thing that all the turns between the interstate and the state park are signed; otherwise, finding the park would have been difficult. The campground is ideal for tent campers. Its nice bathhouse and two disabled-access campsites, 19 and 20, are immediately adjacent to the walk-in parking area. A hilltop field backs the parking area, and a foot trail takes you to the balance of the campsites.

The foot trail leads toward Lake James. Tulip trees and other hardwoods shade the peninsula jutting into the deeply colored water. Reach campsites 1, 2, and 3 on the perimeter of a small knob where the campground woodyard stands. Pine and locust trees shade these sites, two of which are cut into a hill.

Another trail circles down to the lake and the lakeside campsites. Site 4 is on a scenic point overlooking the lake. Shortoff and Table Rock mountains are easily visible in the distance. A wood fence borders the site along the lake, as it is a good 20 feet off a bluff down to the water. A walking trail continues to the rest of the sites. Site 5 is long and narrow. Site 6 overlooks the lake and is shaded by pines. Site 7 is on the small side. Site 8 is highly coveted for its views. Site 9 is 30 feet back from the lake and is cut into the mountainside. Site 10 has numerous landscaping timbers that tier down to the lake itself, where a tiny beach overlooks a cove. Site 11 is back from the water a bit, while site 12

RATINGS

Beauty: ✿ ✿ ✿ ✿ ✿
Privacy: ✿ ✿ ✿
Spaciousness: ✿ ✿ ✿
Quiet: ✿ ✿ ✿
Security: ✿ ✿ ✿ ✿ ✿
Cleanliness: ✿ ✿ ✿ ✿ ✿

is directly on the cove. Site 13, smallish and shaded by white pines, is close to site 14. The water laps up to site 15. Site 16 is in a small flat. Site 17 is near an old foundation with steps leading to the lake. Site 18 is ideal for solitude seekers, set back in the woods all by itself with a path leading only to it.

Water spigots are adequately spaced throughout the area, with few sites spaced over a large area. Trails lead back toward the campground bathhouse. The campground fills on good-weather weekends from late spring until Labor Day. Sites are available through the week anytime the campground is open.

Many campers use this as a base camp to explore western North Carolina, from Linville Gorge and the Blue Ridge Parkway to Asheville and the Biltmore Hotel. Other campers remain within the confines of the park. Still others just hang around their campsites.

Lake James comprises 6,510 acres of alluring water and has 150 miles of shoreline, 5 miles of which are within the park. The swim beach is popular with tent campers during the summer (expect the water to be a tad cooler than that of your average lake). Canoes are available for rent during the summer.

Those with boats will be launching at one of two nearby ramps to explore a few acres of water and a few miles of shoreline. The cool, deep waters harbor largemouth and smallmouth bass, bream, and walleye. Hiking trails are a bit limited at this small state park. One leads a half mile to Sandy Cliff Overlook, where you can enjoy more lake and mountain vistas. A 1.5-mile path leads from the campground to Lake Channel Overlook. The Fox Den Trail is the park's longest, at 2.2 miles. An information board at the walk-in parking area will get you oriented. Hopefully, you will orient yourself and your tent to the lake-view, walk-in sites at Lake James State Park.

KEY INFORMATION

ADDRESS:	P.O. Box 340 Nebo, NC 28761
OPERATED BY:	North Carolina State Parks
INFORMATION:	(828) 652-5047; ncparks.gov; reservations: (877) 722-6762
OPEN:	March 15– November 30
SITES:	20
EACH SITE:	Picnic table, fire ring, lantern post, tent pad
ASSIGNMENT:	First come, first served and by reservation
REGISTRATION:	Ranger will come by to register you
FACILITIES:	Hot showers, water spigots
PARKING:	At walk-in tent parking only
FEE:	$15
ELEVATION:	1,240 feet
RESTRICTIONS:	*Pets:* On leash only *Fires:* In fire rings only *Alcohol:* Prohibited *Vehicles:* None *Other:* 14-day stay limit

MAP

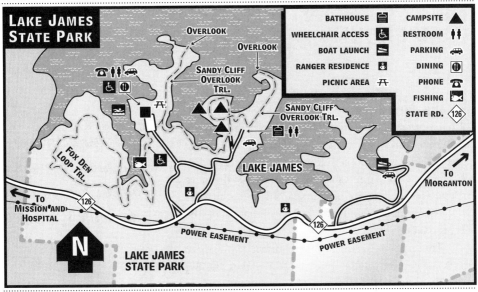

LAKE JAMES STATE PARK

OVERLOOK

OVERLOOK

SANDY CLIFF OVERLOOK TRL.

SANDY CLIFF OVERLOOK TRL.

FOX DEN LOOP TRL.

LAKE JAMES

To MORGANTON

To MISSION AND HOSPITAL

POWER EASEMENT

POWER EASEMENT

N

LAKE JAMES STATE PARK

BATHHOUSE		CAMPSITE	
WHEELCHAIR ACCESS		RESTROOM	
BOAT LAUNCH		PARKING	
RANGER RESIDENCE		DINING	
PICNIC AREA		PHONE	
		FISHING	
		STATE RD.	126

GETTING THERE

From Exit 90 on I-40 west of Morganton, leave north from the interstate, taking Fairview Road 0.4 miles to Harmony Grove Road. Turn right on Harmony Grove Road, and follow it 2.1 miles to reach US 70. Turn left on US 70 west, and follow it 0.2 miles to reach NC 126 east. Turn right on NC 126 east and follow it 2.7 miles to the state park, on your left.

GPS COORDINATES

UTM Zone (WGS84) 17S

Easting 0418570

Northing 3954430

Latitude 35 43' 56.3"

Longitude 81 53' 59.8"

9
LAKE POWHATAN CAMPGROUND

Asheville

LAKE POWHATAN is a nicely developed, well-maintained recreation destination. While it is a great destination in its own right, its proximity to Asheville adds the possibilities of visiting tourist destinations in the area, such as the grand Biltmore Estate. Hikers, mountain bikers, and lake enthusiasts will also find much to like about this slice of the Pisgah National Forest.

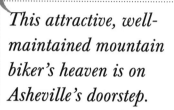

This attractive, well-maintained mountain biker's heaven is on Asheville's doorstep.

The groomed campground is divided into three loops situated on wooded hills above the lake. The Big John Loop has 21 sites—mostly shaded by a pine, oak, and hickory forest—and it is the highest of them all. Each site has been leveled with landscaping timbers, despite the hilliness. Large and attractive, the sites here provide ample privacy. The Bent Creek Loop has sites 22 through 35. It also has hilly, large camps with rich woods. All the sites here are in great condition. The Lakeside Loop, with sites 36 through 57, is actually well above Lake Powhatan, though a few of the sites overlook the water. The sites here are the shadiest, sheltered by hemlock trees.

The Hardtimes Loop, with sites 58 through 97, is my favorite. It's older than the others and looks a little more worn, yet is well kept. This least-used loop, set on a ridgeline rife with dogwoods, actually has two loops. There are many attractive sites to choose from; you just have to be a little pickier. You will enjoy the pretty forest up here.

The campground is gated and manned with hosts who help keep the place in good, clean shape. Water spigots are conveniently set throughout. All the loops except Bent Creek have showers, but Bent Creek does have a restroom. Lake Powhatan can and does fill on summer holidays, but a reservation system can assure you of a campsite whenever you desire. Take advantage of it.

RATINGS

Beauty: ✿ ✿ ✿ ✿
Privacy: ✿ ✿ ✿ ✿
Spaciousness: ✿ ✿ ✿ ✿ ✿
Quiet: ✿ ✿ ✿ ✿
Security: ✿ ✿ ✿ ✿ ✿
Cleanliness: ✿ ✿ ✿ ✿ ✿

ADDRESS:	375 Wesley Branch Rd. Asheville, NC 28806
OPERATED BY:	Pisgah National Forest
INFORMATION:	(828) 670-5627; cs.unca.edu/nfsnc; reservations: (877) 444-6777, recreation.gov
OPEN:	May–October
SITES:	97
EACH SITE:	Picnic table, fire ring, lantern post; most sites have tent pads
ASSIGNMENT:	First come, first served and by reservation
REGISTRATION:	At entrance station
FACILITIES:	Hot showers, flush toilets
PARKING:	At campsites only
FEE:	$18
ELEVATION:	2,100 feet
RESTRICTIONS:	*Pets:* On leash only *Fires:* In fire rings only *Alcohol:* At campsites only *Vehicles:* No more than two per site *Other:* 14-day stay limit, 30-day annual limit

Bent Creek was dammed to form Lake Powhatan, an impoundment that is attractive to both swimmers and anglers. One side of the lake has a large beach and swimming area, while the other side has a fishing pier. The lake is stocked with rainbow, brook, and brown trout, and you can also fish Bent Creek. No boats are allowed on the lake.

A network of hiking and mountain-biking trails weaves out from Lake Powhatan. The whole area is within the confines of the Bent Creek Research and Demonstration Forest. On the way in you will pass several national forest mountain-biking trailheads. Here you can make loops aplenty in the greater Bent Creek watershed, including up Wolf Creek, Ledford Branch, and Boyd Branch. Milder nature trails head directly out of the campground; one track circles the lake. Deerfield Loop and Pine Tree Trail let you explore the woods without getting in your car. The former winds through a variety of ecosystems surrounding Lake Powhatan; the latter has interpretive information that helps you understand the forest through which you walk. Homestead Loop is a short trail that passes over Lake Powhatan Dam. You do have to get in your car, but it is a short distance to visit the North Carolina Arboretum, which you will pass on your way in. Stop at the visitor center to learn more about this outdoor learning center.

Asheville is just a few miles up I-26; you'll find all manner of activities there.

The national forest offers interpretive programs between Memorial Day and Labor Day. Many of these are tailored to kids of all ages, so you can keep junior busy while you can get that much-needed R&R time.

MAP

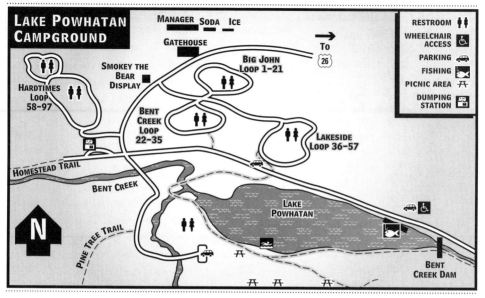

LAKE POWHATAN CAMPGROUND

MANAGER   SODA   ICE

GATEHOUSE

To [26]

SMOKEY THE BEAR DISPLAY

BIG JOHN LOOP 1-21

HARDTIMES LOOP 58-97

BENT CREEK LOOP 22-35

LAKESIDE LOOP 36-57

HOMESTEAD TRAIL

BENT CREEK

N

PINE TREE TRAIL

LAKE POWHATAN

BENT CREEK DAM

RESTROOM
WHEELCHAIR ACCESS
PARKING
FISHING
PICNIC AREA
DUMPING STATION

GETTING THERE

From Exit 33 on I-26 south, take NC 191 south 2 miles to the signed right turn at a traffic light. Keep forward on Wesley Branch Road to dead-end into the campground.

GPS COORDINATES

UTM Zone (WGS84)	17S
Easting	0352540
Northing	3927730
Latitude	35 29' 0.6"
Longitude	82 37' 30.7"

10
LINVILLE FALLS CAMPGROUND

Linville Falls lies at the head of the rugged Linville Gorge Wilderness.

THE BLUE RIDGE PARKWAY is an unusual national park. It is linear, stretching 469 miles on the spine of the Southern Appalachians, connecting the Great Smoky Mountains and Shenandoah national parks. When deciding to designate the first national park in our southern mountains, government officials just couldn't decide between Shenandoah and the Smokies, so both were developed. As a result of this compromise, the scenic road connecting them was built. In the process, officials brought many historic sites and attractive natural features under the park-service umbrella. One of these outstanding areas is Linville Falls, the crown jewel of Linville Gorge, which many consider the most scenic wilderness in the Tar Heel State.

Linville Falls Campground, just off the parkway, can be your base for exploring the gorge. This campground is fairly large, with 70 sites, 50 of which are for tent campers. Oddly, the tent and trailer sites are inter-mixed along two paved camping loops with paved pullins. The setting, at 3,200 feet in elevation, is a flat alongside the clean, clear Linville River. A mixture of white pine, hardwoods, rhododendron, and open grassy areas allows campers to choose the amount of sun and shade they want. Along Loop A are several appealing tent sites set in the woods directly riverside.

On the B Loop are two groupings of tent sites beneath beech trees. Your best bet is to cruise the loops and look for the site that most appeals to you. A sizable grassy meadow is free of campsites and makes for a great sunning or relaxing spot. The biggest drawback to the campground is its mixed placement of tent and trailer campsites. Nonetheless, choosy tent campers will be able to find a good spot. Water spigots are scattered about the campground, and the two bathroom facilities are located within easy walking distance of all the sites. For your

RATINGS

Beauty: ✪ ✪ ✪
Privacy: ✪ ✪ ✪
Spaciousness: ✪ ✪ ✪ ✪
Quiet: ✪ ✪ ✪
Security: ✪ ✪ ✪ ✪ ✪
Cleanliness: ✪ ✪ ✪ ✪ ✪

safety and convenience, campground hosts and park personnel are on-site in the warm season. During winter, the water is turned off and vault toilets are used.

Linville Falls is your mandatory first destination. The falls, in two sections, drop at the point where the Linville River descends into its famous gorge. A park visitor center near the campground is your departure point. The Erwins View Trail is a 1.6-mile round trip that takes hikers by four overlooks, passing the upper and lower falls. The Upper Falls View comes first. You can see both falls from Chimney View. The Gorge View allows a look down into the deep swath cut by the Linville River as it descends between Linville Mountain and Jonas Ridge. Erwins View offers an even more expansive vista than the previous three. Another hike leads steeply from the visitor center down to the Plunge Basin, at the base of the falls. To access the main gorge, managed under the auspices of the U.S. Forest Service, campers must drive a short distance to Wisemans View Road and the Kistler Memorial Highway, a scenic auto destination rivaling the Blue Ridge Parkway. Below, the Linville Gorge Wilderness covers nearly 11,000 acres. Wisemans View is particularly scenic, allowing visitors to gaze up the gorge. Hikers have to trace steep and challenging trails to reach the river down in the gorge, and I know firsthand that they're pretty tough once you are in the gorge. A trail map of the gorge is available at the parkway visitor center. Bynum Bluff Trail makes a sharp drop down to a sharp bend in the river. Babel Tower Trail ends at a locale encircled by the Linville River on three sides. Before taking off on any of these trails, you might want to get a hearty meal at the nearby Linville Falls community, where you can also buy limited camping supplies.

KEY INFORMATION

ADDRESS:	199 Hemphill Knob Rd. Asheville, NC 28801
OPERATED BY:	National Park Service
INFORMATION:	(704) 298-0398; nps.gov/blri; reservations: (877) 444-6777, recreation.gov
OPEN:	April–October
SITES:	50 tent sites, 70 total
EACH SITE:	Picnic table, fire grate, grill
ASSIGNMENT:	First come, first served and by reservation
REGISTRATION:	At campground entrance booth
FACILITIES:	Water spigot and flush toilets
PARKING:	At campsites only
FEE:	$16, additional fee for reserving sites
ELEVATION:	3,200 feet
RESTRICTIONS:	*Pets:* On 6-foot or shorter leash *Fires:* In fire grates only *Alcohol:* At campsites only *Vehicles:* 30-foot trailer-length limit *Other:* 14-day stay limit, 30 days per year

MAP

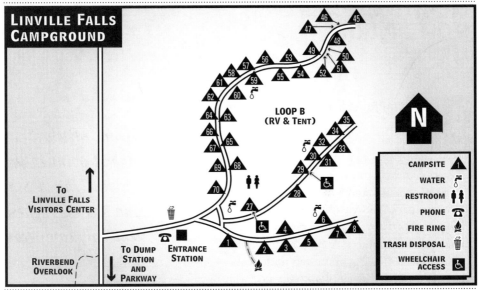

LINVILLE FALLS CAMPGROUND

LOOP B
(RV & TENT)

To
LINVILLE FALLS
VISITORS CENTER

RIVERBEND
OVERLOOK

To DUMP
STATION
AND
PARKWAY

ENTRANCE
STATION

CAMPSITE	▲
WATER	
RESTROOM	
PHONE	☎
FIRE RING	
TRASH DISPOSAL	
WHEELCHAIR ACCESS	♿

GETTING THERE

From Spruce Pine, drive east on NC 226 6 miles to the Blue Ridge Parkway. Head north on the parkway 12 miles to milepost 316.3 and Linville Falls. The campground will be on the right.

GPS COORDINATES

UTM Zone (WGS84) 17S
Easting 0415630
Northing 3981140
Latitude 35 58' 22.1"
Longitude 81 56' 8.9"

11
MOUNT MITCHELL STATE PARK

BRING WARM CLOTHES with you to Mount Mitchell. The rarefied air up here calls to mind Canada more than Dixie. The flora and fauna follow suit. Luckily, in 1915, then-North Carolina Governor Locke Craig recognized the special character of this mountaintop and made it North Carolina's first state park. Now, with a tent-only campground and some superlative highland scenery, Mount Mitchell State Park is a Southern Appalachian highlight.

As the last Ice Age retreated north, cold-weather plants and animals of the north retreated with them—except for those that survived on the highest peaks down in Dixie. These mountaintops formed, in effect, cool-climate islands where the northern species continue to survive. Unfortunately, the mountaintop is under siege by acid rain, insect pests, and a severe climate. As a result, some trees and plants are dying.

Mount Mitchell's campground is for tents only, unless you can carry an RV from the parking area up the stone steps to the campground. The short walk immediately enters the dense forest once dominated by the Fraser fir. Today, stunted and weather-beaten mountain ash and a few other hardwoods mingle with the firs. Dead trees remind you of the trouble these forests face.

The nine campsites splinter off the gravel path that rises with the mountainside. Set into the land amid the dense woods, they are small and fairly close together, but are private due to the heavy plant growth. There is little canopy overhead, as the trees become gnarled the higher they grow. Two water spigots lie along the short path; a bathroom with flush toilets is midway along the path. Firewood is sold by the bundle in the parking area.

Sites 1 and 9 are the most private, but you'll feel lucky to get a site at all during summer weekends. This

> *Mount Mitchell is the highest point in the eastern United States and has the highest tent-only campground.*

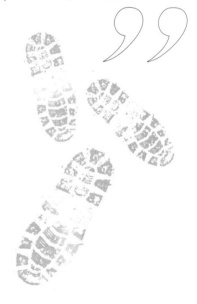

RATINGS

Beauty: ✿ ✿ ✿ ✿ ✿
Privacy: ✿ ✿ ✿ ✿
Spaciousness: ✿ ✿ ✿
Quiet: ✿ ✿ ✿ ✿
Security: ✿ ✿ ✿ ✿ ✿
Cleanliness: ✿ ✿ ✿ ✿ ✿

KEY INFORMATION

ADDRESS: 2388 NC 128
Burnsville, NC
28714

OPERATED BY: North Carolina
State Parks

INFORMATION: (828) 675-4611;
ncparks.gov;
reservations:
(877) 722-6762

OPEN: Year-round; full
facilities May 1–
October 31

SITES: 9 primitive

EACH SITE: Tent pad, grill,
picnic table

ASSIGNMENT: First come,
first served and
by reservation

REGISTRATION: Ranger will come
by to register you

FACILITIES: Water, flush
toilets

PARKING: At tent campers'
parking area only

FEE: $15, $9 in winter

ELEVATION: 6,320 feet

RESTRICTIONS: *Pets:* On 6-foot or
shorter leash
Fires: In fire grates
only
Alcohol: Not
allowed
Vehicles: None
Other: No gather-
ing of firewood in
the park; 14-day
stay limit

tiny campground exudes an intimate, secluded feel. The only noise you'll hear is the wind whipping over your head. By the way, Mount Mitchell is covered in fog, rain, or snow 8 out of every 10 days. Snow has been recorded every month of the year; 104 inches fall annually. Don't let those facts deter you, though—weather is part of the phenomenon that is Mount Mitchell.

The fog rolled in and out of the campground during our midsummer trip. Now and then the sun would shine, warming us. Wooded ridges came in and out of view with the fog; the whole scene seemed like some other world.

Carry a jacket along when you tramp the park. First drive up to the summit parking area, and make the short jaunt to the observation tower atop Mount Mitchell. Here lie the remains of Elisha Mitchell, who fell to his death from a waterfall after measuring the height of the mountain. From the tower you can see the Black Mountain Range and beyond. Back near the parking area, check out the museum that details the natural history of Mount Mitchell.

Many hiking trails thread the park. From the campground you can walk to the observation tower and connect to the Deep Gap Trail; it's a rugged 6-mile hike along the Black Mountain Range to several peaks that stand more than 6,000 feet high. Or you can leave the campground on the Old Mount Mitchell Trail past the park restaurant and loop around Mount Hallback to return to the campground.

Mount Mitchell State Park is surrounded by the Pisgah National Forest, which is bisected by the Blue Ridge Parkway. This, in essence, increases the accessible forest area beyond the 1,860-acre state park. Many national forest trails connect to the state park trails, allowing nearly unlimited hiking opportunities. Procure a trail map from the park office for the best hiking experience.

Get your supplies in Asheville before you leave. Also check for the latest road conditions on the parkway at nps.gov/blri. The Blue Ridge Parkway makes for a scenic drive, but once in the highlands of the Black Mountains, you won't want to leave this wonderful mountaintop and campground.

MAP

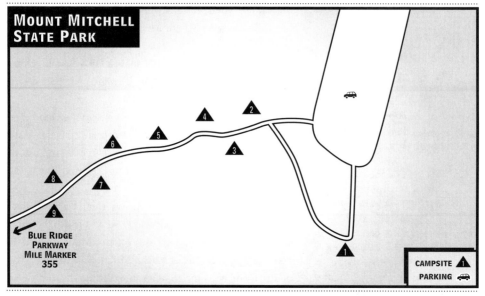

MOUNT MITCHELL
STATE PARK

8

9

7

6

5

4

2

3

1

BLUE RIDGE
PARKWAY
MILE MARKER
355

CAMPSITE ▲
PARKING 🚗

GETTING THERE

From Asheville, take the
Blue Ridge Parkway north
34 miles to milepost 355.
Turn left into Mount
Mitchell State Park. The
campground is 4 miles up
the road on your right.

GPS COORDINATES

UTM Zone (WGS84) 17S
Easting 0385000
Northing 3957630
Latitude 35 45' 27.5"
Longitude 82 16' 20.3"

12
MOUNT PISGAH CAMPGROUND

Loops exclusively for tent campers complement the natural beauty of this nearly mile-high campground.

THIS IS THE HIGHEST CAMPGROUND on the entire Blue Ridge Parkway at nearly 5,000 feet. And that is just the beginning of the superlatives here. Try secluded sites just for tent campers in a high-country forest, complete with stately spruce trees. How about nature trails circling the campground? Throw in some new hot showers added to the comfort stations. Add some fantastic views along the parkway, and you have a great tent-camping destination.

The campground is wonderfully integrated into the mountain landscape of greater Mount Pisgah, specifically just below Flat Laurel Gap, amid the headwaters of Pisgah Creek and the 85-acre Flat Laurel bog, a rare high-country wetland where wind-sculpted birch and maple trees shade the campsites. Rhododendron and mountain laurel grow in dense thickets that offer plenty of privacy. Evergreens tower above all other vegetation. In this woodland, four different loops put like-minded campers together. Loop A is for RVs but is little used by RVs or tent campers. Loop B is for pop-ups and campers, so it doesn't have tent pads, and the sites are less level than Loops C and D. Loop B has hot showers, as does Loop C.

Loops C and D are designated tent-camping loops, with 32 and 36 sites, respectively. Their tent sites are cut out of the forest, with heavy vegetation between them. Sometimes steps lead up or down to the sites from the paved auto pull-ins. If you have to look for a complaint, the sites are a tad small, and a few in C are a little close to the parkway. Overall, the sites are well maintained and well groomed, which adds to the already beautiful natural scenery.

Campsites are available without reservations any time except the major summer holiday weekends, but reservations can be made at any time. A campground host keeps things safe and orderly. Be apprised that

RATINGS

Beauty: ☆ ☆ ☆ ☆ ☆
Privacy: ☆ ☆ ☆ ☆
Spaciousness: ☆ ☆ ☆
Quiet: ☆ ☆ ☆ ☆
Security: ☆ ☆ ☆ ☆
Cleanliness: ☆ ☆ ☆ ☆

food-storage regulations are in effect as a safeguard against bears. Because this campground is high, be prepared for cool conditions whenever you come.

The Blue Ridge Parkway sets the tone for Mount Pisgah, and you will enjoy great scenery on the way in. Once at the campground, you can enjoy walking some of the nature trails that form a network through and around the campground. Head to the tower atop Frying Pan Mountain, or loop over to Buck Spring Gap then walk to the top of Mount Pisgah, at 5,721 feet.

Not enough hiking opportunities? Why don't you visit Shining Rock Wilderness, just a few miles south on the Blue Ridge Parkway? I've enjoyed trekking here among the open fields, rock outcrops, and forests of this high-country preserve. Middle Prong Wilderness is less visited, more remote, and more wooded. Yellowstone Prong, a stream near Graveyard Fields Overlook south of the campground, has loop trails leading to three different falls, all relatively close together. The Cradle of Forestry Visitor Center is just a few miles down US 276 toward Brevard; see where the science of forestry began and explore some of the nature trails here. If you want to get wet, head down to Sliding Rock, a water feature on Looking Glass Creek where people shoot down a natural water slide into a pool. It's fun if you've never done it. Finally, the Mountains-to-Sea Trail traverses more miles along this area of the parkway than most hikers want to hike. A trail map of the Pisgah District of the Pisgah National Forest, which surrounds the parkway, comes in very handy here.

From the campground, a trail leads to the camp store, which sells some supplies and is near the Pisgah Inn on the other side of the parkway from Mount Pisgah. The inn serves breakfast, lunch, and dinner in case you don't feel like cooking. And you may be too tired to cook after all the hiking around here.

KEY INFORMATION

ADDRESS:	199 Hemphill Knob Rd. Asheville, NC 28803
OPERATED BY:	National Park Service
INFORMATION:	(828) 298-0398; nps.gov/blri; reservations: (877) 444-6777, recreation.gov
OPEN:	Mid-May–late October
SITES:	68 tent sites, 29 pop-up and van sites, 33 RV sites
EACH SITE:	Picnic table, fire grate, lantern post; some sites have tent pads
ASSIGNMENT:	First come, first served and by reservation
REGISTRATION:	At campground kiosk
FACILITIES:	Hot showers, flush toilets, water spigots
PARKING:	At campsites only
FEE:	$16, plus additional fee if reserving site
ELEVATION:	4,980 feet
RESTRICTIONS:	*Pets:* On leash only *Fires:* In fire rings only *Alcohol:* At campsites only *Vehicles:* No more than two per site *Other:* 21-day stay limit

MAP

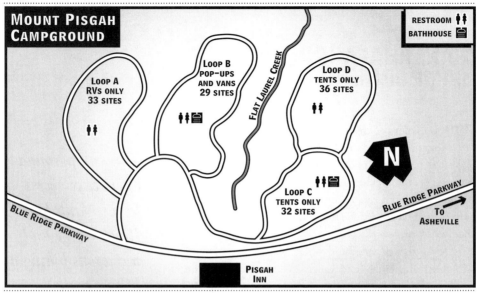

MOUNT PISGAH CAMPGROUND

RESTROOM 👫
BATHHOUSE 🛁

LOOP B
POP–UPS
AND VANS
29 SITES

FLAT LAUREL CREEK

LOOP D
TENTS ONLY
36 SITES

LOOP A
RVs ONLY
33 SITES

👫🛁

👫

N

LOOP C
TENTS ONLY
32 SITES

👫🛁

BLUE RIDGE PARKWAY
To
ASHEVILLE

BLUE RIDGE PARKWAY

PISGAH
INN

GETTING THERE

From Asheville, take I-26
south to Exit 33/NC 191.
Take NC 191 south to the
Blue Ridge Parkway and
milepost 393.6; then turn
south and take the parkway
to milepost 408. The campground will be on your right.

GPS COORDINATES

UTM Zone (WGS84) 17S
Easting 0340480
Northing 3919110
Latitude 35 24' 16.9"
Longitude 82 45' 23.9"

13
NELSON'S NANTAHALA HIDEAWAY CAMPGROUND

The owners of this facility knew they had a good location from which tent campers could access the numerous outdoor features in the immediate vicinity, so they set about creating a good campground to match the first-rate scenery of the area. They're still working out a few kinks, but you'll be more than satisfied with your stay here.

Pass the campground office, which has ice and soft-drink machines, and enter the campground. The design features the classic loop, which climbs up the side of a hill along a small creek, Powder Burnt Branch. The campsites are set along tiers that extend from one side of the loop to the other. This lets campers enjoy topographic relief without having to camp on a slope, as the tiers are level and evenly graded. The lower end of the loop is more open.

Several generations ago, the campground was a cornfield; later, trees reclaimed the site. When the campground was built, the many trees were left to flourish and naturally landscape Nelson's Hideaway. Tree cover thickens as the campground rises, with a thick carpet of grass forming the understory.

The centrally located bathhouse is simply the finest I've ever seen this side of a fancy hotel, much less a campground. Divided by gender, each attractive section contains three hot showers and flush toilets enclosed within a rustic wood exterior. Wash your dirty duds at the laundry facility, located here as well. Water spigots are spread throughout the campground.

If you don't feel like pitching a tent, use one of the Adirondack-style, open-air shelters at the beginning of the loop. They have padded bunks and a small porch where you can enjoy the cool mountain breezes. Each shelter has a picnic table beside it. Three sizable group campsites, in a flat across Powder Burnt Branch, can be reached by crossing a small footbridge.

> *This campground offers easy access to the Nantahala River Gorge and numerous biking and hiking trails.*

RATINGS

Beauty: ☆ ☆ ☆
Privacy: ☆ ☆ ☆
Spaciousness: ☆ ☆ ☆ ☆
Quiet: ☆ ☆ ☆ ☆
Security: ☆ ☆ ☆ ☆ ☆
Cleanliness: ☆ ☆ ☆ ☆ ☆

ADDRESS: P.O. Box 25
US 19/74
Topton, NC 28781

OPERATED BY: Jimmy Kyle Davis

INFORMATION: (800) 936-6649 or
(828) 321-4407;
nantahalacamp
ground.com

OPEN: Mid-April–
October

SITES: 30

EACH SITE: Tent area, picnic
table, fire ring

ASSIGNMENT: First come, first
served and by
reservation

REGISTRATION: At campground
office

FACILITIES: Water, hot
showers, laundry,
soft-drink
machine, some
electrical hookups

PARKING: At campsites only

FEE: $20 per night; $30
per night for three
or more persons

ELEVATION: 2,800 feet

RESTRICTIONS: *Pets:* On leash only
Fires: In fire rings
only
Alcohol: At camp-
sites only
Vehicles: None

Tent campers seek out the top of the loop, where the woods thicken and campers are kings of the hill. You can see across the valley to the Snowbird Mountains.

The middle tiers are equipped with electricity in addition to the regular amenities. But don't expect too many RVs here: It's a steep climb to the campground from the highway. In addition, with all the hiking, canoeing, and kayaking opportunities, active campers are likely to be found here.

Just 2 miles north is the Nantahala River Launch Site. Here, canoeists and kayakers enter the river gorge for a 9-mile run of nationally known white-water floating. Commercial outfitters will accommodate inexperienced thrill seekers who long to challenge the chilly, continuous rapids.

The Nelson family has built hiking trails on its land that connect to the Apple Tree national forest trails that border the campground. This is only fitting, since earlier family generations actually sold the Apple Tree land to the federal government to form a section of the Nantahala National Forest. The trails follow old routes that connected Cherokee lands in western North Carolina and eastern Tennessee.

The London Bald Trail is closest to the campground property. Reached from Piercy Creek, this trail connects to the Laurel Creek and Diamond Valley trails, providing numerous loop-hiking opportunities. Also, the Bartram National Scenic Trail is easily reached via the London Bald Trail. Consult the campground office for a hiking map.

Adjacent to the campground is a cool, clear fishing pond. An old-fashioned waterwheel oxygenates the water, where trout thrive. For stream fishing, head to nearby Piercy Creek. Nantahala Lake is just a few miles east for lake-fishing possibilities. An assortment of mountain-biking trails threads the nearby national forest land, which nearly envelops the campground.

Combine the fine new facilities of Nelson's Nantahala Hideaway with the recreational variety of this section of western North Carolina, and you have a successful tent-camping adventure.

MAP

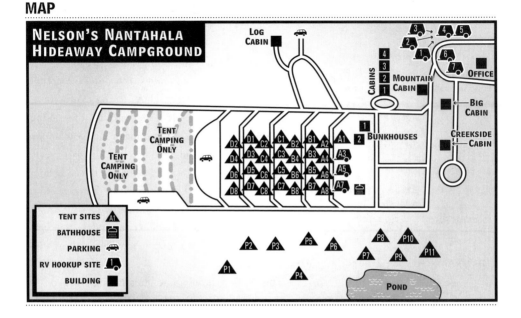

NELSON'S NANTAHALA HIDEAWAY CAMPGROUND

LOG CABIN

MOUNTAIN CABIN

CABINS

OFFICE

BIG CABIN

CREEKSIDE CABIN

TENT CAMPING ONLY

TENT CAMPING ONLY

D2 D1 C2 C1 B2 B1 A2 A1

D4 D3 C4 C3 B4 B3 A4 A3

D6 D5 C6 C5 B6 B5 A6 A5

D8 D7 C8 C7 B8 B7 A8 A7

BUNKHOUSES

TENT SITES A1
BATHHOUSE
PARKING
RV HOOKUP SITE 1
BUILDING

P2 P3 P5 P6 P8 P10

P1 P7 P9 P11

P4

POND

GETTING THERE

From Andrews, take US 19/74 north 6 miles to the community of Topton. Nelson's Nantahala Hideaway will be on your right.

GPS COORDINATES

UTM Zone (WGS84)	17S
Easting	0254000
Northing	3903330
Latitude	35 14' 40.8"
Longitude	83 42' 12.1"

14
NEW RIVER
STATE PARK

This tent campground on the banks of the New River is one of the best in the state.

NORTH CAROLINA IS BLESSED with many rivers, some of which are so exceptional as to receive wild and scenic designation. The New River is one of these. Located in the most northwesterly portion of the state, the New River courses through the mountains, northbound for Virginia. The state of North Carolina has long recognized the New River's beauty and works to protect this natural treasure while making it accessible, with canoe access points and campgrounds such as New River State Park. The riverside sites are all walk-in, or boat-in if you are traveling overnight down the river. No matter how you arrive, you will agree that this tent campground situated on the banks of the New is one of the best in the state.

Leave the walk-in parking area and cross a mown field, passing the remains of an old homestead with the chimney still standing. Reach campsite 9, sitting all alone in a small flat beside the spring run of the old homesite. Beyond here, the forest is regenerating in formerly plowed fields. A mix of black walnut, locust, and tulip trees shades the area amid thick brush. Mown paths reach the sites. Site 8 is circled by brush and shaded by cherry trees. Cross a little wet-weather stream to enter the rest of the campground. Site 7 is directly along the river and is shaded by walnut trees. Site 6 is also along the river, but a steep bank prevents direct river access—the campground operates its own river landing, and park personnel encourage using only this access to keep down erosion. Site 5 is adjacent to campsite 6.

Site 4 is on a slight slope, but landscaping timbers have been added to level it beneath crab apple trees. Site 3 is closest to the bathhouse, which is heated in the cooler months. Shaded by tulip trees and located beside the campground's river access, site 2 is the most

RATINGS

Beauty: ✿ ✿ ✿ ✿
Privacy: ✿ ✿ ✿ ✿
Spaciousness: ✿ ✿ ✿ ✿
Quiet: ✿ ✿ ✿ ✿ ✿
Security: ✿ ✿ ✿ ✿
Cleanliness: ✿ ✿ ✿ ✿

popular, especially with boat-in campers. Site 1 is also near the boat access but is farther into the woods and is heavily shaded.

This campground at the Wagoner Access fills on holiday weekends only. It can get a little busy at the beginning and end of summer. Sites are always available on weekdays. Critters such as raccoons abound in this area, so secure your food while camping here.

Most folks who camp here like to paddle the river, but even if you're not a boater, you can still have a good time. The mile-plus Fern Nature Trail circles the valley beside the campground. Add a mile and connect with the Running Cedar Trail. A pretty picnic area, once an apple orchard, lies adjacent to the camping area. The trees still produce fruit, attracting deer and humans alike in fall. A rapid drops just above the campground access, offering fishing opportunities and a decent little swimming hole below it. A large field below the parking area affords room for games and general running around.

But face it: This park was developed with the paddler in mind. The state manages 26 miles of river here and maintains several access points for day and overnight trips. A popular run here is from the NC 88 bridge down to Wagoner Access, 5 miles in length. From Wagoner Access to the US 221 Access is 11 miles; plan for an all-day trip. Paddling times vary with river flows and weather conditions. Also, trips run slower if you like to fish your way downriver, as I do. Angling here is good for smallmouth bass, rock bass, and bream. Determined anglers might land a muskie.

An outfitter is located nearby if you are boatless or just want a shuttle. Zaloo's Canoes offers inner tubes for fun, canoes for rent, and shuttle services of varying lengths. Reservations are required. For more information, call (800) 535-4027 or visit **zaloos.com.** The river scenery is both mountainous and pastoral, deserving of its wild and scenic status. Rapids are mild, not exceeding Class 2, making the New a great training river. After you enjoy the Wagoner Access on the river, you'll want to check out other state park access areas that lie along this preserved water in North Carolina's northwest corner.

KEY INFORMATION

ADDRESS:	P.O. Box 48 Jefferson, NC 28640
OPERATED BY:	North Carolina State Parks
INFORMATION:	(336) 982-2587; ncparks.gov; reservations: (877) 722-6762
OPEN:	Year-round
SITES:	9
EACH SITE:	Picnic table, fire grate, trash can
ASSIGNMENT:	First come, first served and by reservation
REGISTRATION:	Ranger will come by to register you
FACILITIES:	Hot showers, flush toilets, water spigots
PARKING:	At lot below ranger station
FEE:	$9
ELEVATION:	2,600 feet
RESTRICTIONS:	*Pets:* On leash only *Fires:* In fire rings only *Alcohol:* Prohibited *Vehicles:* None *Other:* 14-day stay limit in a 30-day period

THE BEST IN TENT CAMPING CAROLINAS

MAP

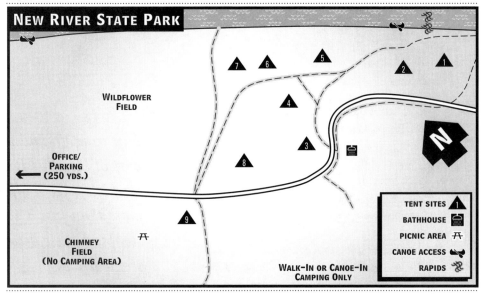

NEW RIVER STATE PARK

WILDFLOWER FIELD

OFFICE/ PARKING
← (250 YDS.)

CHIMNEY FIELD
(NO CAMPING AREA)

WALK-IN OR CANOE-IN CAMPING ONLY

TENT SITES
BATHHOUSE
PICNIC AREA
CANOE ACCESS
RAPIDS

GETTING THERE

From the junction with US 421 on the west side of Wilkesboro, take NC 16 north 23 miles to NC 88. Turn right, heading east on NC 88, and follow it 1.4 miles to Wagoner Access Road. Turn left on Wagoner Access Road, and follow it 1 mile to enter the park.

GPS COORDINATES

UTM Zone (WGS84) 17S
Easting 0465420
Northing 4029860
Latitude 36 24' 54.7"
Longitude 81 23' 8.5"

HIGH IN THE FORESTS of the Blue Ridge Mountains, Julian Price Memorial Park offers good camping and plenty of activities that don't involve an automobile. Don't let the size of the campground scare you off. There are nearly 200 sites in three areas: one area for RV camping only, one for one-night camping only, and another for both RV and tent camping.

The one-night-only camping loop backs against the shores of Price Lake. The south end of the paved loop is thickly forested, both overhead and on the ground, for maximum privacy. Five sites are right along the lakeshore. The other end of the loop circles a field and is more open. A few pull-through RV sites are here. A lighted bathroom is conveniently placed at the center of the loop for all campers to share. Two water spigots are located at each end of this spacious, private loop.

The main RV and tent area has three loops. Loops C and D spur off the larger Loop B. Oddly enough, Loop D is actually inside Loop B; Loop C spurs off on its own. All are in a rolling woodland and are set into the mountains without dominating the natural landscape. The plethora of trees overhead reminds you that you are in the forest. The rhododendron understory provides plenty of privacy; however, it isn't everywhere, which means you can move about the campground freely. Landscaping timbers were used where site leveling was necessary. Some of the sites in Loops B and C are a tad close together, but with investigating and luck, you can find a private site. Nine water spigots are scattered throughout these three loops for easy water access, and three lighted bathrooms ensure that you never have to go too far if nature calls in the middle of the night.

Loops E and F are for RVs only and concentrate these campers in one location. On my visit to Price Park, I didn't see any other RVers outside of E or F,

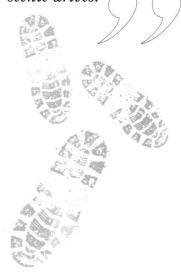

This campground is part of the Blue Ridge Parkway, yet it offers more than just a stopping place between scenic drives.

RATINGS

Beauty: ☆ ☆ ☆ ☆ ☆
Privacy: ☆ ☆ ☆
Spaciousness: ☆ ☆ ☆ ☆
Quiet: ☆ ☆ ☆ ☆
Security: ☆ ☆ ☆ ☆
Cleanliness: ☆ ☆ ☆ ☆ ☆

KEY INFORMATION

ADDRESS:	199 Hemphill Knob Rd. Asheville, NC 28801
OPERATED BY:	National Park Service
INFORMATION:	(828) 298-0398; nps.gov/blri
OPEN:	Mid-May– October 31
SITES:	129
EACH SITE:	Tent pad, picnic table, fire grate, lantern post
ASSIGNMENT:	First come, first served; no reservations
REGISTRATION:	Register at campground check-in station
FACILITIES:	Water, flush toilets, pay phone; concessions sold on main road in spring and summer
PARKING:	At campsites only
FEE:	$16
ELEVATION:	3,400 feet
RESTRICTIONS:	*Pets:* On 6-foot or shorter leash *Fires:* In fire grates only *Alcohol:* At campsites only *Vehicles:* 30-foot trailer-length limit *Other:* 14-day stay limit, 30-day total limit for calendar year

with the exception of a couple in the one-night-only loop. Expect a full house on hot summer weekends, when nearby lowlanders escape the heat. A ranger and a campground host reside at the campground to answer questions and ease your safety concerns.

Even the most ardent auto tourists have to stretch their legs every once in a while and see for themselves just what is beyond the roadside. Price Park offers the Blue Ridge sightseer plenty to do outside the car. Trails run through the campground, which makes starting a hike even easier.

The Boone Fork Trail makes a 5-mile loop passing through many environments of the Blue Ridge. It leaves the campground to enter a meadow and picks up an old farm road. It then runs along Bee Tree Creek, crossing it 16 times. Pass through a rocky area and return to the campground through a meadow.

The 2.3-mile Green Knob Trail climbs to an overlook that will reward you with well-earned views of Price Lake, then loops back via Sims Pond. The Tanawha Trail runs 13 miles south along the Blue Ridge Parkway and obviously requires a shuttle. A segment of the nearly complete North Carolina Mountains-to-Sea Trail passes through Price Park on its way to the Atlantic.

The Price Lake Trail makes a 2.3-mile loop around the 47-acre lake, which contains three species of trout that you can angle for: rainbow, brook, and brown. Nearby Sims Pond has only the native brook trout. Stream anglers can try Boone Fork and Sims Creek for trout as well. A valid North Carolina fishing license is required.

During the 1940s, Julian Price bought this area as a retreat for his company employees. His heirs willed the area to the National Park Service for all of us to enjoy. As scenic as the Blue Ridge Parkway is, you may find this special area hard to pass. Stop and spend a day enjoying the sights with no glass between you and nature.

MAP

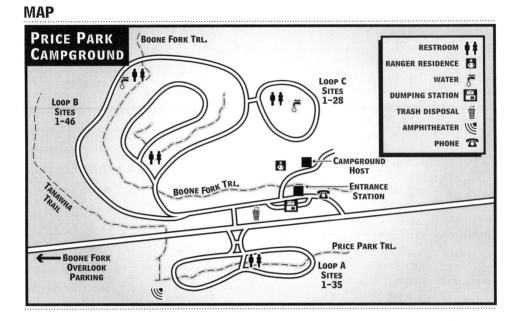

PRICE PARK CAMPGROUND

BOONE FORK TRL.

LOOP C
SITES
1-28

LOOP B
SITES
1-46

TANAWHA TRAIL

BOONE FORK TRL.

CAMPGROUND
HOST

ENTRANCE
STATION

BOONE FORK
OVERLOOK
PARKING

PRICE PARK TRL.

LOOP A
SITES
1-35

RESTROOM	👫
RANGER RESIDENCE	🏠
WATER	🚰
DUMPING STATION	🚽
TRASH DISPOSAL	🗑
AMPHITHEATER	📢
PHONE	☎

GETTING THERE

From Boone, take US 321 east 7 miles to the Blue Ridge Parkway. Turn south on the parkway, and follow it 7 miles to Julian Price Memorial Park. The campground check-in station will be on your right.

GPS COORDINATES

UTM Zone (WGS84) 17S
Easting 0433550
Northing 3999460
Latitude 36 8' 21.9"
Longitude 81 44' 18.4"

16
ROCKY BLUFF CAMPGROUND

The design of this campground will capture your fancy, and the setting will make you stay.

AS I HEADED DOWN into the Rocky Bluff Recreation Area, I found it hard to believe that there was a campground there. The road dipped into hilly terrain, with nary a flat spot to be found. But soon enough, there was the beginning of Rocky Bluff Campground. "Engineering marvel" may be a stretch, but a ton or two of site leveling and stonework were necessary to fit this campground into the wooded dips and rises of the land. All that stonework makes your back ache just looking at it.

Rocky Bluff Campground is divided into two loops. Enter the lower loop as you pass the pay station. Three shaded sites are dug into the hillside and reinforced with the above-mentioned stonework. Five open sites sit on the inside of the loop, on what passes for flat ground here at Rocky Bluff.

At the low point of the lower loop, a road spurs off to the right and leads to the upper loop. As the road makes a steep climb, two campsites are somehow fit into the terrain. Seven sites lie on top of the hill, spread along the road as it makes a short loop to return to the main campground. Two sites offer a view into Spring Creek hollow to the east.

A warning to those who get spooked easily: Also atop this hill, right next to the campsites, is Brooks Cemetery. Three sites look on to it. Stay down on the lower loop if the proximity of the cemetery will prevent you from enjoying a sound night's sleep.

Intersect the lower loop again from the upper-loop road. Here, sites are strewn in the open, lightly wooded center of the loop; a few more are tucked away in the thickets outside the loop. There isn't a whole lot of privacy. Due to the sloping terrain, you are probably going to be looking down on another camper or vice versa. A generally grassy understory doesn't shield you much from your neighbor, either. The upper loop,

RATINGS

Beauty: ✿ ✿ ✿ ✿
Privacy: ✿ ✿ ✿
Spaciousness: ✿ ✿ ✿
Quiet: ✿ ✿ ✿ ✿
Security: ✿ ✿ ✿
Cleanliness: ✿ ✿ ✿ ✿

where ironically you might want to keep your neighbor in view to make sure he isn't a ghost roaming from the cemetery, is more wooded.

The lower-loop road passes a picnic area on the right and returns to the pay station. This loop has the only comfort station for the 30-site campground. Those on the upper loop must walk down the hill to use the facilities. But water spigots are conveniently placed around both loops for your convenience.

This campground is neat. The terrain and stone-work make it unique, and the cemetery adds a touch of history and mystique. If the cemetery isn't enough of the past, imagine this place a century ago when there was a community of homes, a blacksmith shop, and a school.

The nearest community, Hot Springs, embodies small-town Appalachia. It's full of nice people who work hard for a living in the splendor of a land that is now more precious to them than ever before. The Appalachian Trail runs right through town. Visit the Pisgah National Forest Visitor Center, and check out the hot springs for which the community was named.

Outdoor pastimes are plentiful. Several outfitters in town will arrange a white-water-rafting trip down the French Broad River, which flows through Hot Springs. A 6-mile biking trail runs along the river to Paint Rock, which marks the Tennessee–North Carolina state line. This dividing line crosses the bridge over the French Broad from Hot Springs. The Appalachian Trail crosses this bridge too. Hike either way on the trail until your legs wear out. Then soothe your muscles in the actual hot springs, but you must pay for the privilege.

Two fulfilling trails depart from Rocky Bluff Campground. The 1.2-mile Spring Creek Nature Trail loops down to Spring Creek and follows it a good way before veering north and intersecting the campground again, making for a rewarding and short day hike. The Van Cliff Loop Trail is a little longer and tougher. It leaves the campground and climbs, crossing NC 209 on the way and hooking up into some piney woods before returning to the campground after 2.6 miles.

KEY INFORMATION

ADDRESS:	P.O. Box 128 Hot Springs, NC 28743
OPERATED BY:	U.S. Forest Service
INFORMATION:	(828) 622-3202; cs.unca.edu/nfsnc
OPEN:	May 1–October 31
SITES:	30
EACH SITE:	Tent pad, fire grate, lantern post, picnic table
ASSIGNMENT:	First come, first served; no reservations
REGISTRATION:	Self-registration on site
FACILITIES:	Water, flush toilets
PARKING:	At campsites only
FEE:	$8
ELEVATION:	1,780 feet
RESTRICTIONS:	*Pets:* On 6-foot or shorter leash *Fires:* In fire grates only *Alcohol:* At camp-sites only *Vehicles:* 18-foot trailer-length limit *Other:* 14-day stay limit

MAP

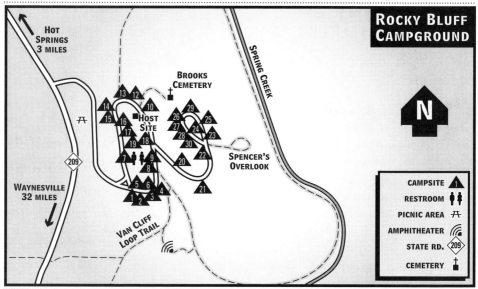

HOT SPRINGS 3 MILES

WAYNESVILLE 32 MILES

ROCKY BLUFF
CAMPGROUND

BROOKS
CEMETERY

SPRING CREEK

HOST SITE

SPENCER'S
OVERLOOK

VAN CLIFF
LOOP TRAIL

N

CAMPSITE	1
RESTROOM	👫
PICNIC AREA	🪑
AMPHITHEATER	🎧
STATE RD.	209
CEMETERY	✝

GETTING THERE

From Hot Springs, take
NC 209 south 3 miles.
Rocky Bluff Campground
will be on your left.

GPS COORDINATES

UTM Zone (WGS84) 17S
Easting 0333880
Northing 3971580
Latitude 35 52' 33.3"
Longitude 82 50' 25.4"

17
SMOKEMONT CAMPGROUND

SMOKEMONT IS STRATEGICALLY located on the Oconaluftee River at the base of the Smoky Mountains. From this location, campers can enjoy the immediate beauty of Great Smoky Mountains National Park and jump onto Newfound Gap Road northbound to explore other segments of the park. Take Newfound Gap Road just a few miles south, and you are in the tourist town of Cherokee. And if that isn't enough, you can take a ride on the Blue Ridge Parkway, which has just come 400-plus miles from Shenandoah National Park in Virginia to end near Smokemont. But this campground, nestled in a flat along Bradley Fork near the Oconaluftee River, exudes an old-time national-park camping atmosphere that may keep you mostly at your campsite, poking a stick into the fire, watching the trees grow, or listening to the water flow.

The campground is much longer than wide, stretching up the hollow of Bradley Fork, a fine, clear mountain stream that serenades the entire campground. Pass the ranger station and campground office. Campsites are strung out in loop form beneath the shade of oaks, maples, dogwoods, and hemlocks. The first loops, A, B, and C, are open year-round, whereas D and F, the RV loops, may be closed in colder times.

Overall, the sites are on the small side, and a lack of brush between campsites limits privacy. Strategically placed river boulders keep cars and campers separated. Old stone outbuildings house the bathrooms and also have outdoor sinks on them for washing dishes. Continue up the hollow to reach D Loop, which has more hemlocks. The sites are situated three wide here; the ones in the middle have less privacy. Shade is extensive throughout the campground and will be welcome in summer. Loop F is across Bradley Fork.

Summer is the busy time. Reservations are available

> *Enjoy the Carolina side of the Smokies while conveniently located near the town of Cherokee.*

RATINGS

Beauty: ✰ ✰ ✰ ✰
Privacy: ✰ ✰
Spaciousness: ✰ ✰ ✰
Quiet: ✰ ✰ ✰
Security: ✰ ✰ ✰ ✰ ✰
Cleanliness: ✰ ✰ ✰ ✰

KEY INFORMATION

ADDRESS:	107 Park HQ Rd. Gatlinburg, TN 37738
OPERATED BY:	Great Smoky Mountains National Park
INFORMATION:	(865) 436-1200; nps.gov/grsm; reservations: (877) 444-6777, recreation.gov
OPEN:	Year-round
SITES:	96, plus 46 RV-only sites
EACH SITE:	Picnic table, fire grate, lantern post; some sites have tent pads
ASSIGNMENT:	First come, first served and by reservation May 15–October 31
REGISTRATION:	At campground entrance station
FACILITIES:	Flush toilets, water spigots, pay phone
PARKING:	At campsites only
FEE:	$17, plus additional fee if reserving site
ELEVATION:	2,200 feet
RESTRICTIONS:	*Pets:* On 6-foot leash only *Fires:* In fire rings only *Alcohol:* At campsites only *Vehicles:* No more than two per site *Other:* 7-day stay limit May 15–October 31; 14-day stay limit November 1–May 14

between May 15 and October 31, so make them if you can. Campsites are available the rest of the year, and people do camp here year-round, even in the depths of winter. A word to the wise: Store your food properly here—this is bear country.

Simply being in the Smoky Mountains is the attraction. There is so much to see in the park. However, there is plenty to do right here in Smokemont, especially hiking. The Smokemont Loop Trail leads along Bradley Fork, then upward along the southern reaches of Richland Mountain and past the Bradley Cemetery, returning to the campground after 5 miles. The Bradley Fork Trail heads toward Cabin Flats, a backcountry campsite that makes a great day-hiking destination along upper Bradley Fork. If you are feeling aggressive, make a loop using Chasteen Creek Trail and head to the high country along Hughes Ridge; then return via Bradley Fork, a good trout-fishing stream. Speaking of fishing, here's a tip—the farther you get from the campground, the better the fishing. Oconaluftee River offers roadside trout angling. Or you can head up Big Cove Road or down into Cherokee for some ramped-up put-and-take fishing on Native American lands. The waters of the Smokies are not just for fishing, however. The cool streams are also good for a summer dip or even tubing. Be careful of slippery rocks and strong currents, though.

As previously mentioned, the Blue Ridge Parkway is good for an auto tour, or you can head up Newfound Gap Road and then onward to Clingmans Dome, the highest point in the park at 6,642 feet. It has a tower for observation. Stop for a visit at the park's Oconaluftee Visitor Center and see the pioneer buildings.

If you want a little touristy fun, head down to Cherokee, where you can buy some moccasins, get some taffy, or gamble at the reservation casino. If you're feeling cultural, check out the outdoor drama *Unto These Hills,* which is held nightly. Arts and crafts abound in town as well. For more info, visit **cherokee-nc.com.** Just remember that you have some camping to do, too, at Smokemont.

MAP

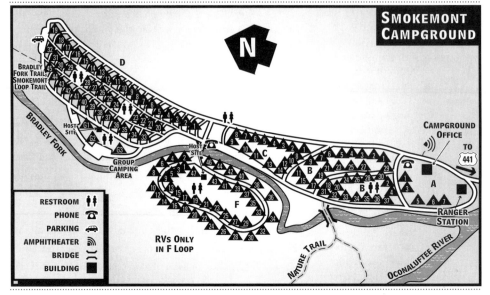

SMOKEMONT CAMPGROUND

N

BRADLEY FORK TRAIL, SMOKEMONT LOOP TRAIL

D

BRADLEY FORK

HOST SITE

GROUP CAMPING AREA

HOST SITE

C

F

B

A

CAMPGROUND OFFICE

TO 441

RANGER STATION

NATURE TRAIL

OCONALUFTEE RIVER

RVs ONLY IN F LOOP

RESTROOM
PHONE
PARKING
AMPHITHEATER
BRIDGE
BUILDING

GETTING THERE

From Cherokee, take Newfound Gap Road, US 441, 3.1 miles beyond the Oconaluftee Visitor Center to the right turn over the Oconaluftee River. Immediately turn left after crossing the river to reach the campground.

GPS COORDINATES

UTM Zone (WGS84) 17S
Easting 0200450
Northing 3937101
Latitude 35 33' 25.9"
Longitude 83 18' 43.1"

18
STANDING INDIAN CAMPGROUND

> *Soak in the mountains of the Standing Indian Basin from the headwaters of the Nantahala River.*

ACCORDING TO CHEROKEE LEGEND, a warrior was once posted on top of a certain mountain to look out for a flying monster that had snatched a child from a nearby village. The villagers prayed to the Great Spirit to annihilate the monster. A violent storm struck the mountain, reducing it to rock and turning the lookout warrior into a stone "standing Indian."

The Nantahala River is born on Standing Indian Mountain just upstream from this outstanding high-country campground, where cool breezes from the ridgetops temper the warm summer air. With sites on five loops, Standing Indian is spread out and offers a variety of site conditions. The first loop diffuses along the Nantahala with hemlock-shaded sites isolated by thick stands of rhododendron. Across the river, three loops are spread out in a large, flat area interspersed with large hardwoods that allow plenty of sun and grass to flourish among their ranks. Ritter Lumber Company once had a logging camp here. Farther back still, across Kimsey Creek, are mountainside sites. They stand level among the sloping forest of yellow birch, beech, and sugar maple, and are separated by lush greenery that makes each site seem isolated. Six double sites accommodate larger groups.

Campground hosts occupy each loop for your safety and convenience. Sixteen water pumps are strategically located throughout the loops, in addition to five comfort stations with flush toilets (two of the comfort stations also have hot showers). There are no electric hookups. You may pick up dead, downed firewood from the surrounding area without a permit. Keep in mind that Standing Indian can be crowded during peak summer weekends.

There's plenty to do nearby. Try your luck at one of the campground horseshoe pits. Fish for trout on the Nantahala River or Kimsey Creek. Rainbow and brown

RATINGS

Beauty: ✿ ✿ ✿ ✿ ✿
Privacy: ✿ ✿ ✿ ✿
Spaciousness: ✿ ✿ ✿ ✿ ✿
Quiet: ✿ ✿ ✿
Security: ✿ ✿ ✿ ✿
Cleanliness: ✿ ✿ ✿ ✿

trout are the predominant cold-water fish in the streams, with some brook trout in the upper waters. For the non-fishing water lover, there are two falls nearby. Drive 5 miles on Forest Service Road 67 beyond the turnoff to the campground. The Big Laurel Falls Trail sign is on the right. After passing over a footbridge, the trail splits. Veer to the right and come to Big Laurel Falls in 0.5 miles. The Mooney Falls Trail starts 0.7 miles beyond the Big Laurel Falls trailhead and leads 0.1 mile to the cascading falls.

Several trails begin at the campground. To orient yourself, find the Backcountry Information Center 0.2 miles left of the campground entrance gate. Study the map. Make an 8-mile loop out of the Park Creek and Park Ridge trails. The Park Creek Trail starts at the Backcountry Information Center; follow it down the Nantahala, then up Park Creek to Park Gap. Take the Park Ridge Trail 3.2 miles back down to the campground. This hike is moderate to strenuous, with a net elevation change of 880 feet.

The most prominent trail in the area is the famed Appalachian Trail, which skirts the campground to the south and east. The 87-mile section extending from the Georgia line to the Smokies is considered by many hikers to be one of the most rugged sections, with its relentlessly steep ups and downs. This section weeds out many thru-hikers who aspire to "follow the white blaze" 2,100 miles to Maine.

The Appalachian Trail passes by FS 67 on the way to the campground. Drive out of the campground toward Wallace Gap about a mile. The Rock Gap parking area is on your right. Take the trail south (uphill to your right), and soon you'll come to the Rock Gap backcountry shelter, one of a series of shelters located about a day's walk from one another along the entirety of the trail. They provide a haven from the elements for the weary thru-hiker. Imagine this as your home for a six-month journey up the spine of the Appalachians.

While you're at Standing Indian Campground, why not see the mountain for which it was named? It's a strenuous 3.9-mile climb to the 5,499-foot peak, but the views provide ample reward. Use the Lower Ridge Trail, which starts on the left just beyond the campground

KEY INFORMATION

ADDRESS:	90 Sloan Rd. Franklin, NC 28734
OPERATED BY:	U.S. Forest Service concessionaire
INFORMATION:	(828) 524-6441; cs.unca.edu/nfsnc
OPEN:	April–November
SITES:	84
EACH SITE:	Tent pad, fire grate, lantern post, picnic table
ASSIGNMENT:	First come, first served; no reservations
REGISTRATION:	Self-registration on site
FACILITIES:	Drinking water, flush toilets, hot showers, phone
PARKING:	At campsites only
FEE:	$14
ELEVATION:	3,400 feet
RESTRICTIONS:	*Pets:* On a leash only *Fires:* In fire grates only *Alcohol:* At campsites only *Vehicles:* 21-foot trailer-length limit; $2 parking at picnic area *Other:* Sites limited to one family or five persons; 14-day stay limit from Memorial Day to Labor Day, 30-day limit otherwise

MAP

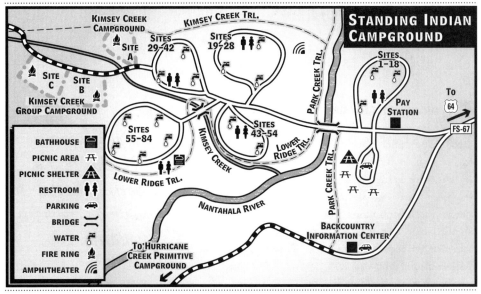

GETTING THERE

From Franklin, drive west on US 64 9 miles to old US 64. Following the sign to Standing Indian, turn left and go 1.5 miles to Wallace Gap. Turn right at the sign on Forest Service Road 67 leading to the campground.

bridge over the Nantahala. Switch back up to the ridge crest, and follow it southward to the Appalachian Trail. Take a spur trail 0.2 miles to the top of Standing Indian, and view the Blue Ridge Mountains and the Tallulah River Basin.

GPS COORDINATES

UTM Zone (WGS84) 17S
Easting 0269190
Northing 3883790
Latitude 35 4' 19.7"
Longitude 83 31' 51.0"

19 SOUTH MOUNTAINS STATE PARK

DURING MY ROAMING while writing this book, park rangers and others kept mentioning South Mountains State Park as an ideal candidate for inclusion here. By the time I got to the park, my expectations were as high as an Appalachian peak. And my trip here was as satisfying as a view from such a high place. South Mountains State Park delivers in both its small, rustic streamside campground and its 18,000 acres of wilderness to explore. This is a wilderness park—nothing but you and nature. After you set up camp, your exploration can be a day trip by foot or mountain bike, or a backpack for those inclined to overnight in the backcountry. Many visitors mix up a trip, first camping in the campground, then setting off into the backcountry. The park's amenities have been carefully integrated into the South Mountains, an outlier range far from the more-popular peaks straddling the North Carolina–Tennessee border.

> *Tent campers will love this rugged backwoods state park with an emphasis on wilderness.*

The 11-site campground is set in a flat along Jacob Fork, a crystalline, musical trout stream that tumbles over gray rocks and resonates among the campsites. Immediately reach campsite 1, where landscaping timbers delineate each site and corral small gravel within the tent pads for drainage. Each site's "fittings," that is, picnic tables and lantern posts, are in fine condition. Tall, straight tulip trees and white pines shade the campground, along with hemlock, sourwood, hickory, maple, and sweetgum. Site 2 is across the campground road from Jacob Fork. Sites 3 and 4 are near the creek and back up against mountain laurel and rhododendron. More sites are set directly along the creek. Site 7 is a handicap-accessible site and has a wide picnic table. Site 8 has many hemlocks overhead. I wish I had stayed in site 9, which backs directly against the stream and overlooks a steep hillside. Site 10 is also beside Jacob Fork. Unfortunately, I arrived just at dark and didn't

RATINGS

Beauty: ✩ ✩ ✩ ✩ ✩
Privacy: ✩ ✩ ✩
Spaciousness: ✩ ✩ ✩
Quiet: ✩ ✩ ✩ ✩
Security: ✩ ✩ ✩ ✩ ✩
Cleanliness: ✩ ✩ ✩ ✩

ADDRESS: 3001 South
Mountains State
Park Ave.
Connelly Springs,
NC 28612

OPERATED BY: North Carolina
State Parks

INFORMATION: (828) 433-4772;
ncparks.gov;
reservations:
(877) 722-6762

OPEN: Year-round

SITES: 11

EACH SITE: Picnic table, fire
ring, lantern post,
tent pad

ASSIGNMENT: First come,
first served and
by reservation

REGISTRATION: Ranger will come
by to register you

FACILITIES: Vault toilets,
water spigots

PARKING: At campsites only

FEE: $9

ELEVATION: 1,350 feet

RESTRICTIONS: *Pets:* On leash only
Fires: In fire rings
only
Alcohol: Prohibited
Vehicles: Trailers of
25 feet or less
recommended
Other: 14-day stay
limit

want to bother other campers by driving through the campground multiple times, even though I normally "loop the loop" before choosing a site. Site 11, the last in the lineup, was my choice. A modern vault toilet and water spigot are conveniently close to this one.

I enjoyed being deep in this mountain valley. So do others, as the small campground fills most summer weekends; I recommend fall or spring, when it's wide open. During spring the wildflowers will be blooming and the creeks running high, which makes the many waterfalls and cascades more enticing. In fall, the colors will be every bit as good as those in the main Appalachian Range, but less busy. Campers can get a site any time of year during the week.

The South Mountains range from 1,200 to around 3,000 feet high. That makes visiting them more appealing in spring and fall, as they will be less chilly than other, higher ranges. Summer can be warm but is not oppressively hot. The park has 40 miles of trails to explore, ranging from a 0.75-mile interpretive nature trail along Jacob Fork, very worth your time, to loops long enough for you to bring your sleeping bag should you attempt them. Popular day hikes are to High Shoals Falls, which can be made into a loop hike, to Little River Falls, and to Jacob Knob Overlook. A good park-trail map reveals other loop possibilities. The many park streams offer trout fishing in an attractive setting. Not only does the park contain the entire Jacob Fork watershed, but it also has acquired the Clear Creek and Henry Fork drainages. Anglers are limited only by time and desire. Be apprised of the latest license requirements and fishing regulations before you strike out.

Mountain bikers have an 18-mile designated loop that the park deems strenuous, so be prepared for an all-day outing on this path, which circles the ridgelines along Jacob Creek—and bring your water bottle. After my experience at South Mountains State Park, I will be circling back to this place for more of the best in tent camping.

MAP

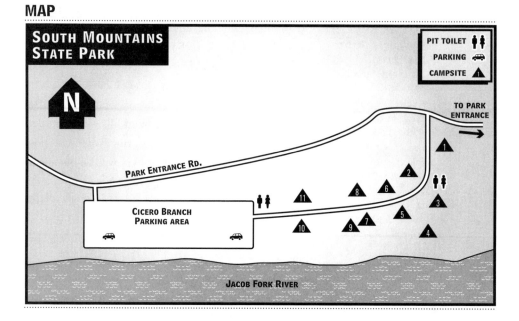

GPS COORDINATES

UTM Zone (WGS84) 17S

Easting 0443530

Northing 3939230

Latitude 35 35' 49.5"

Longitude 81 37' 23.8"

GETTING THERE

From Exit 105 on I-40 near Morganton, take NC 18 south 11 miles to Sugar Loaf Road. Turn right on Sugar Loaf Road and follow it 2 miles; then turn left on Old NC 18 Road. Take Old NC 18 Road 2.6 miles; then turn right on NC 1901 (Wards Gap Road), follow it 1.3 miles, and veer right onto South Mountains Park Road. Follow South Mountains Park Road 3.5 miles to reach the campground.

> *Head straight from the tent and go mountain biking, boating, horseback riding, hiking, or fishing.*

WHAT DO A CHEROKEE, a pioneer, a big dam, and mountain biking have in common? Answer: They have all played a major part in the evolution of Tsali Recreation Area.

In 1838, during a forced removal of native peoples to the American West that became known as the Trail of Tears, a Cherokee leader by the name of Tsali turned himself in so other Cherokee could remain in the area. These natives formed the nucleus of the Eastern Band of Cherokee, who now live on a reservation adjacent to Bryson City. Early in this century, pioneer Harv Brown raised corn along Mouse Branch; there he turned his grain into "corn juice," otherwise known as moonshine. In the 1940s, when Fontana Dam was built, Harv and his kinfolk moved away. Now Harv's plot is Tsali Campground, where hikers, horseback riders, and especially mountain bikers congregate. These hearty adventurers catch their collective breath here at Tsali between excursions along the 39 miles of trails that emanate from the campground bordering Fontana Lake.

Tsali Campground is divided into two loops, an upper and a lower. The upper loop has 22 sites. The U.S. Forest Service keeps the campground well groomed, and plenty of second-growth hardwoods and pines shade the former field. A sparse understory makes the campground open yet sacrifices privacy. Six of the sites are spread along Mouse Branch. Four water spigots are evenly dispersed along the loop. In its center sit a pair of low-volume flush toilets.

The lower loop features 19 sites and is more open and spacious than the upper loop, having fewer trees and, in some spots, a grassy understory. Eight sites back against Mouse Branch. At the head of the lower loop is a modern bath facility with flush toilets and hot showers, which are quite popular with sweaty hikers and bikers. Three water spigots are conveniently

RATINGS

Beauty: ✫ ✫ ✫ ✫
Privacy: ✫ ✫ ✫
Spaciousness: ✫ ✫ ✫
Quiet: ✫ ✫
Security: ✫ ✫ ✫ ✫ ✫
Cleanliness: ✫ ✫ ✫ ✫ ✫

located on this loop, where a short trail leads down to Fontana Lake.

The campground is full on weekends and busy during the week with active campers. Mountain bikers from all over the Southeast converge on Tsali to ride its trails. Many campers bring canoes as well, to drift on Fontana Lake and glide on the nearby white-water rivers. Hikers abound; pleasure boaters and equestrians are represented, too.

There are four primary Tsali trails. The U.S. Forest Service has devised a system enabling hikers, bikers, and equestrians to enjoy the trails without bothering one another. Hikers can use all four trails at any time. The Right Loop and Left Loop trails are paired together. The Mouse Branch and Thompson Loop trails are paired together in a system whereby equestrians and bikers alternate using them daily. Right Loop Trail is a single-track trail that extends for 11 miles with views of Fontana Lake. It can be shortened to 4- or 8-mile loops. The Left Loop Trail is a 12-mile, single-track pathway that features an overlook with a view of the Smoky Mountains. Mouse Branch Trail mixes a single-track trail with old logging roads and passes through old homesites along its 6-mile course. You may see wildlife on the 8-mile Thompson Loop Trail, which crosses streams and passes through wildlife openings and old homesites. Check the trail-use schedule posted at the campground.

The boat ramp presents more recreational opportunities. You can fish in Fontana Lake or access the Smokies. Cross the water and anchor in any cove on the Smokies side of the lake. Then meander up the creek that created the cove, and you will run into the Lakeshore Trail, which runs for miles in both directions. Many relics of the past may be seen, including stone walls, chimneys, and broken china. Make it an adventure. But remember, all artifacts are part of the park and must be left behind for others to enjoy.

Other facilities at Tsali include a bike-washing area for cleaning up after those long, muddy rides; a stable for horses; and a bank-fishing trail near the boat launch for safely wetting a line. If you need supplies, drive west on NC 28 to Wolf Creek General Store.

KEY INFORMATION

ADDRESS:	1131 Massey Branch Rd. Robbinsville, NC 28771
OPERATED BY:	U.S. Forest Service
INFORMATION:	(828) 479-6431; cs.unca.edu/nfsnc
OPEN:	April 14– October 31
SITES:	41
EACH SITE:	Tent pad, lantern post, picnic table, fire grate
ASSIGNMENT:	First come, first served; no reservations
REGISTRATION:	Self-registration on site
FACILITIES:	Water, flush toilets, hot shower
PARKING:	At campsites only
FEE:	$16
ELEVATION:	1,750 feet
RESTRICTIONS:	*Pets:* On leash only *Fires:* In fire rings only *Alcohol:* At campsites only *Vehicles:* None *Other:* 14-day stay limit

MAP

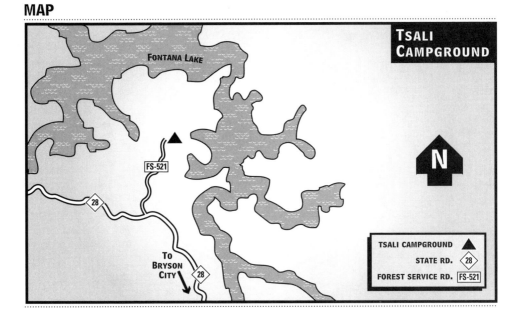

GETTING THERE

From Bryson City, take US 19 south 9 miles. Then turn right on NC 28 5.5 miles. Turn right again at the signed junction on Forest Service Road 521, and follow it 1.5 miles. Tsali Campground will be on your left.

This is a fun area for active people. Use Tsali as a base camp, and enjoy all of the activities available in this beautiful section of the Southern Appalachians.

GPS COORDINATES

UTM Zone (WGS84) 17S
Easting 0264930
Northing 3920950
Latitude 35 24' 21.3"
Longitude 83 35' 11.7"

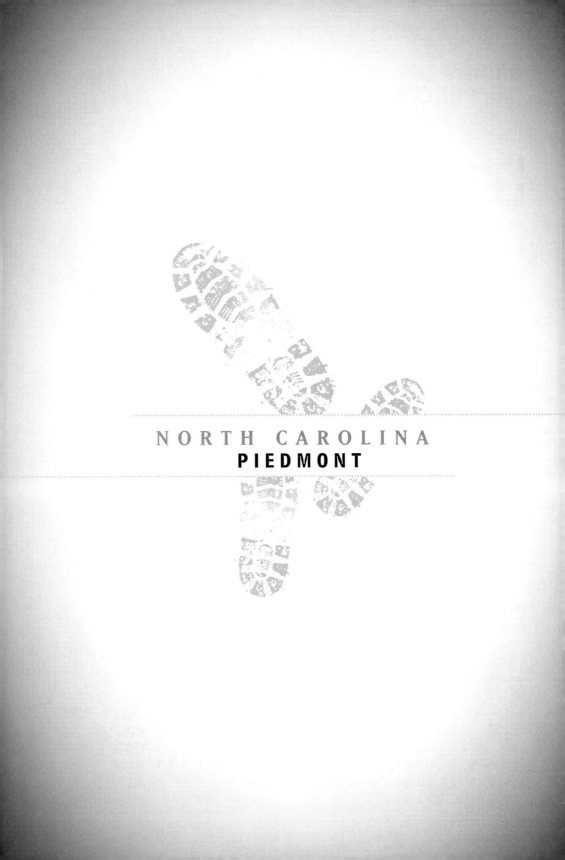

NORTH CAROLINA
PIEDMONT

21
BADIN LAKE
CAMPGROUND

DEPENDING ON WHERE you're coming from, there are several ways to reach Badin Lake Campground. Most of them take a lot of twists and turns, but the drive is worth it. This lakeside campground is the pride of the Uwharrie National Forest and is a best bet for tent campers who want a good campground accompanied by water and land recreation, including boating, fishing, and hiking. Maybe that's why it seems that all roads and signs in the Uwharrie National Forest lead to Badin Lake Campground, which has gotten a recent makeover and now includes hot showers and flush toilets in the bathhouses.

This lakeside camp is broken into two loops. The Lower Loop has campsites 1 through 21. The terrain slopes toward Badin Lake, but the sites themselves have been leveled with landscaping timbers. Some sites are multitiered. Pines reach high, with cedars, oaks, sweetgum, and heavy brush below. The lakeside sites start with 4, which is a double. Other double sites are 13, 20, and 22. If you are reserving a site and want to camp by the lake, go for sites 4, 6, 8, 9, 11, 12, or 13, which are singles. The Lower Loop curves away from the lake and offers more-attractive, wooded sites.

On a hill overlooking the lake, the Upper Loop has sites 22 through 34. This loop is lesser used and offers the most solitude; being farther from Badin Lake makes it less popular. Sites 26 and 29 are closest to the water. All sites are reservable, so crowding isn't a concern if you plan ahead. The sites are generally large and appear to be well maintained. Heavy brush between sites offers more-than-adequate privacy. A campground host is on duty most of the year, providing an element of safety not found at unhosted campgrounds. Both loops have bathhouses with shower facilities.

Badin Lake, covering 5,350 acres, is an impoundment of the Yadkin River. The eastern shore of the lake

> *Badin Lake offers water and land recreation in the Uwharrie Mountains.*

RATINGS

Beauty: ☆ ☆ ☆
Privacy: ☆ ☆ ☆ ☆
Spaciousness: ☆ ☆ ☆
Quiet: ☆ ☆ ☆ ☆
Security: ☆ ☆ ☆ ☆ ☆
Cleanliness: ☆ ☆ ☆ ☆

KEY INFORMATION

ADDRESS: 789 NC Highway 24/27 East Troy, NC 27371

OPERATED BY: U.S. Forest Service

INFORMATION: (910) 576-6391; cs.unca.edu/nfsnc; reservations: (877) 444-6777 or (877) 722-6762, recreation.gov

OPEN: Year-round

SITES: 34

EACH SITE: Picnic table, fire grate, tent pad, lantern post

ASSIGNMENT: First come, first served and by reservation

REGISTRATION: Self-registration on site

FACILITIES: Hot showers, flush toilets, water spigots

PARKING: At campsites only

FEE: $12

ELEVATION: 525 feet

RESTRICTIONS: *Pets:* On leash only *Fires:* In fire rings only *Alcohol:* Prohibited *Vehicles:* None *Other:* 14-day stay limit

borders the national forest and is where the campground is located. Favored fish are bluegill, crappie, largemouth bass, catfish, and stripers. Anglers will be using worms and crickets with a bobber in spring for bluegill. Get on a bed of the slabsiders, and you are in for some fun. Bass will be moving according to season; try looking for them at rocky points or around submerged logs. Crappie generally will go for minnows. Stripers are large bass that can be caught on live shad or top-water lures. Catfish are bottom-feeders and will go for chicken livers or even a hot dog if the bait is kept on the lakebed with weights.

While others ski, swim (although no formal swimming area exists), and sun on the lake, campers with lakeside sites can enjoy the water directly from their tents. For those with boats, Cove Boat Ramp is 2 miles from Badin Lake Campground, near Arrowhead Campground. Badin Lake Campground has a fishing pier nearby if you are boatless. Campers can enjoy lakeside hiking directly from their sites. Badin Lake Trail leads north and south along the shore to a make a loop. Southbound hikers will reach Cove Boat Ramp and Arrowhead Campground after 2.2 miles. The path then returns through the woods to the lake, circling around a north point then curving south past Kings Mountain Point, which also has a fishing pier. If you leave north from Badin Lake Campground, it is only 0.5 miles to Kings Mountain Point. The entire loop is 5.5 miles. You can hike to a remote spot and fish from shore or just look for wildlife, especially birds. Look also for evidence of gold mining, such as pits and tailings. Just realize your richest find here will be your campsite at Badin Lake Campground.

MAP

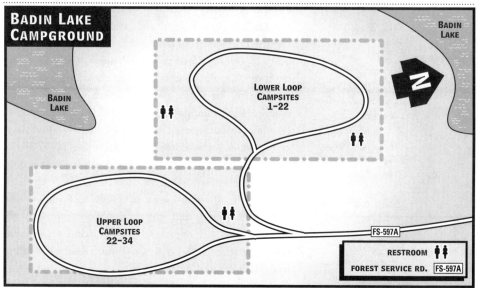

BADIN LAKE CAMPGROUND

BADIN LAKE

BADIN LAKE

LOWER LOOP CAMPSITES 1-22

UPPER LOOP CAMPSITES 22-34

FS-597A

RESTROOM

FOREST SERVICE RD. FS-597A

GPS COORDINATES

UTM Zone (WGS84) 17S

Easting 0583690

Northing 3922860

Latitude 35 26' 51.7"

Longitude 80 4' 40.2"

GETTING THERE

From Troy, head north on NC 109 10 miles to Reservation Road. Make a sharp left onto Reservation Road. Follow it 0.4 miles, then turn right on Moccasin Creek Road. Follow it 0.6 miles, then turn right on McCleans Creek Road/Forest Service Road 544. Turn right on FS 544, and follow it 2.7 miles to Badin Lake Road. Turn right on Badin Lake Road and follow it a short distance; then veer left on FS 597A and follow it to the campground. All these turns are signed.

> *This state park is deservedly popular for its far-reaching vistas and tumbling cascades.*

I CAN UNDERSTAND why Hanging Rock is so popular. The natural setting is dramatic: the Sauratown Mountains rise from the Piedmont in barren rock faces, forming natural vista points for overlooking the surrounding countryside. Hiking trails explore not only mountain lookouts, but also waterfalls and woodlands. A ridge-rimmed lake with recreation opportunities offers a watery contrast to the land. Park facilities include a wood-and-stone bathhouse by the lake that is listed on the National Register of Historic Places. The lodgelike visitor center fits well in the setting and is full of interpretive information about the land, people, and history of this nearly 7,000-acre state park. Finally, the campground is an adequate jumping-off point for getting out and exploring this active camper's destination.

The campground at Hanging Rock is divided into two loops. The first loop has campsites 1 through 42 and is open throughout the week. Hickory, oaks, and maples shade the ridgeline campground, which is slightly sloped. Sourwood, sassafras, and mountain laurel form a thick understory that screens the sites from one another. Sites are situated as the rocks and trees allow, resulting in sites of differing sizes and distances from the loop. A trail leads down to the park lake, which is in the valley below the campground.

The second loop, with sites 43 through 73, is stretched on a ridgeline road. It is open only on weekends. The sites on the right side of the road are more desirable, as they face into the lake valley rather than toward the campground access road. Mountains are visible beyond the lake through the trees. The campground road descends along the ridge, but the sites themselves have been leveled. Be aware that these sites are closer together than those in the first loop.

RATINGS

Beauty: ✰ ✰ ✰ ✰
Privacy: ✰ ✰ ✰
Spaciousness: ✰ ✰
Quiet: ✰ ✰ ✰
Security: ✰ ✰ ✰ ✰ ✰
Cleanliness: ✰ ✰ ✰ ✰

Each loop has a bathhouse. Water spigots are adequately spread throughout the campground, which has a host to make your stay go more smoothly. The only real downside to this park is the popularity of the campground, which fills just about every nice weekend. First come, first served means take your chances, but get here by 1 p.m. on a Friday to get a site. Better yet, try to come during the week, or mix your weekends and weekdays together if you can swing it.

More than 18 miles of trails travel to and through the park's natural features. Hanging Rock Trail leads to the park's namesake. The area on the overhang is rugged and rocky! You can even see downtown Winston-Salem from here. Additional views await at other destinations. An observation tower, once a fire tower used by the state forest service, is at Moore's Knob, where many a passerby has inscribed his or her name in the rock bluff. Check out the vistas from Cook's Wall, which leads to a cliff edge and House Rock. Other worthwhile hiking destinations are the Lower Cascades, Upper Cascades, Window Falls, and Hidden Falls. Haven't gotten enough falls? Then head to Tory's Falls. Here also is Tory's Den, a cave that was purportedly used during the Revolutionary War.

The park lake has a rustic bathhouse built by the Civilian Conservation Corps between 1935 and 1942. A slope leads beyond the bathhouse to a beach, then to the clear lake, which was dammed by the CCC. This attractive impoundment offers fishing from a pier. Visitors can also rent paddleboats and rowboats to tool around the lake or angle for bream and bass (no private boats are allowed, though). The impressive park visitor center has an interesting video from the CCC days, among other information that is worth a visit. As pretty as the park structures may be, the natural landscape is the star of the show here. Make time to pitch your tent, and check it out for yourself.

KEY INFORMATION

ADDRESS:	P.O. Box 278 Danbury, NC 27016
OPERATED BY:	North Carolina State Parks
INFORMATION:	(336) 593-8480; ncparks.gov; reservations: (877) 722-6762
OPEN:	Year-round
SITES:	73
EACH SITE:	Picnic table, fire grate, tent pad
ASSIGNMENT:	First come, first served and by reservation
REGISTRATION:	Ranger will come by to register you
FACILITIES:	Hot shower, flush toilets, water spigot, bathhouse open March 15–November, pit toilet only in winter
PARKING:	At campsites only
FEE:	$15; $9 in winter
ELEVATION:	1,500 feet
RESTRICTIONS:	*Pets:* On leash only *Fires:* In fire rings only *Alcohol:* Prohibited *Vehicles:* Must be on parking pad *Other:* 14-day stay limit in a 30-day period

MAP

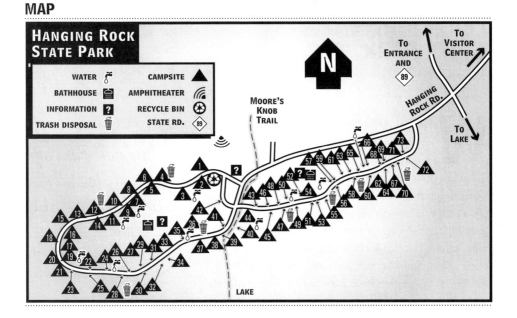

GETTING THERE

From Winston-Salem, take Exit 110B from US 52, and follow US 311 17 miles to NC 89. Keep forward on NC 89 west 9 miles to Hanging Rock Road. Turn left on Hanging Rock Road and follow it 1 mile to enter the state park.

GPS COORDINATES

UTM Zone (WGS84) 17S
Easting 0565260
Northing 4025710
Latitude 36 23' 20.1"
Longitude 80 16' 41.4"

23
LAKE NORMAN
STATE PARK

Troutman

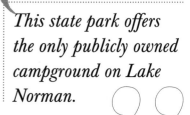

WITH A NAME LIKE LAKE NORMAN, this state park is obviously a water-oriented destination. In that regard, it doesn't disappoint. Nearly the entire preserve is situated on a peninsula jutting into this impoundment, located just north of the greater Charlotte area. So it's no surprise that the park campground is by the water and that the park has a swim area, a boat launch, shore fishing, and a hiking trail that curves along the lake. If that's not enough water, there's more—Lake Norman State Park has its own small lake where you can rent canoes and paddleboats.

> *This state park offers the only publicly owned campground on Lake Norman.*

Once you arrive at the park, it seems to take forever to get to the actual campground. That is because the campground is at the tip of the peninsula that the state park owns. Having only 33 sites keeps the atmosphere relaxed even when the campground is full, which is just about every nice weekend between mid-April and Labor Day. Enter a loop with one crossroad cutting it in half. The peninsula is hilly enough to offer vertical variation, but the campsites have been leveled. A tent pad at each site assures a level night's sleep. Many sites also have leveled picnic-table pads so the camp stew won't tip off your stove. A pretty forest of cedar, shortleaf pine, sourwood, and other hardwoods shades the campground. The forest is young but thick, and it offers good privacy.

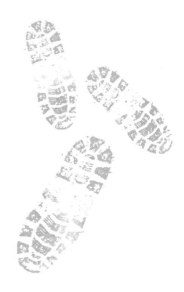

Past the first three sites, the main campground road continues curving along the lakeshore while a crossroad turns left. A connector hiking trail leaves the campground to meet the Lakeshore Trail across from site 3. Sites 4, 5, and 6 are sloped downhill toward the lake and are heavily shaded. Site 12 is closest to the water, but none of the sites are directly lakeside. Sites 13 and 14 jut toward the water but are close to each other. The lake views are gone by site 20. Campsites 23 and 24 offer good solitude. The campground crossroad, on which the

RATINGS

Beauty: ☆ ☆ ☆
Privacy: ☆ ☆ ☆ ☆
Spaciousness: ☆ ☆
Quiet: ☆ ☆
Security: ☆ ☆ ☆ ☆ ☆
Cleanliness: ☆ ☆ ☆

ADDRESS:	159 Inland Sea Ln. Troutman, NC 28166
OPERATED BY:	North Carolina State Parks
INFORMATION:	(704) 528-6350; ncparks.gov; reservations: (877) 722-6762
OPEN:	March 15– November 30
SITES:	33
EACH SITE:	Picnic table, fire ring, tent pad
ASSIGNMENT:	First come, first served; and by reservation
REGISTRATION:	Ranger will come by to register you
FACILITIES:	Hot showers, flush toilets, water spigots
PARKING:	At campsites only
FEE:	$15
ELEVATION:	800 feet
RESTRICTIONS:	*Pets:* On leash only *Fires:* In fire rings only *Alcohol:* Prohibited *Vehicles:* Car must fit on campsite pull-in *Other:* 14-day stay limit

camp host stays, has sites 26 through 33, which are a bit packed in. Site 31 is near the bathhouse, which centers the loop and is convenient to all campers.

The campground as a whole is well maintained and appealing. Plan on getting a site by noon on Friday during high summer. Weekdays aren't crowded, but the area does get some traffic from I-77.

As mentioned earlier, this state park is centered on the water. The swim area on Lake Norman is popular during the summer. Boatless campers can fish from shore or head up to the small park lake, rent a paddleboat or canoe, and fish in a no-gas-motors atmosphere. Those with boats will use the park's boat ramp to access Lake Norman for fishing, skiing, and general water recreation. If you want to be near the water but not on it, take the Lake Shore Trail. It meanders along most of the peninsula, which is bordered by Hicks Creek and the main lake. The entire loop is a 6.5-mile trek. Or take a shortcut on the Short Turn Trail and make your loop only 3.4 miles. The Alder Trail is much shorter, at 0.8 miles. It is located at the park lake, where the rental boats are. This used to be a busier area when the swim beach was here, but it now seems forgotten. Bicyclists love to pedal along the many park roads. There's even a 3-mile mountain-bike trail for those who want a little off-road pedaling action. And there is plenty of outdoor action here at Lake Norman State Park.

MAP

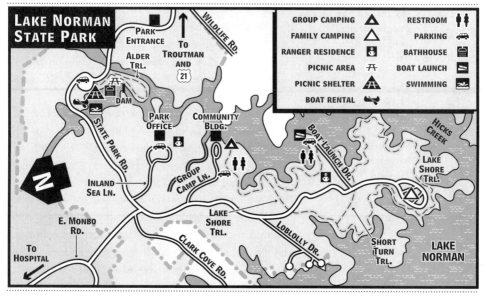

LAKE NORMAN STATE PARK

PARK ENTRANCE
ALDER TRL.
To TROUTMAN AND 21
WILDLIFE RD.

GROUP CAMPING	△	RESTROOM
FAMILY CAMPING	△	PARKING
RANGER RESIDENCE		BATHHOUSE
PICNIC AREA	⊤	BOAT LAUNCH
PICNIC SHELTER	△	SWIMMING
BOAT RENTAL		

DAM
PARK OFFICE
COMMUNITY BLDG.
STATE PARK RD.
BOAT LAUNCH DR.
HICKS CREEK
LAKE SHORE TRL.
INLAND SEA LN.
GROUP CAMP LN.
E. MONBO RD.
LAKE SHORE TRL.
LOBLOLLY DR.
CLARK COVE RD.
SHORT TURN TRL.
LAKE NORMAN
To HOSPITAL

GETTING THERE

From Exit 42 on I-77, just south of Statesville, take US 21 north 2.7 miles to the town of Troutman. Take a sharp left on Perth Road, and follow it 1.5 miles to State Park Road. Turn right on State Park Road, and follow it for 2 miles to enter the park.

GPS COORDINATES

UTM Zone (WGS84) 17S
Easting 0506000
Northing 3947060
Latitude 35 40' 9.2"
Longitude 80 56' 2.8"

24
MORROW
MOUNTAIN
STATE PARK

> *This mountainous get-away on the Piedmont features hiking, boating, fishing, and swimming.*

THE PEAKS OF MORROW MOUNTAIN will surprise you. They aren't the "big highs" of western North Carolina, but if you want a touch and feel of the mountains without having to make the trip west, come here. Relative to the terrain of the surrounding Piedmont, the Uwharrie Mountains rise to offer vertical relief and a mountain aura to the upper Pee Dee River Valley. Back in the 1930s, local residents noted the area's beauty and strove to develop a park. Today the 4,700-acre park offers a large campground, more than 30 miles of trails, and water recreation on Lake Tillery, which is located at the base of the mountains.

Normally a campground with more than 100 sites can resemble a mini–tent city. Morrow Mountain, however, bucks the trend. Three separate loops are spread over a wide area, each with its own bathhouse, giving the impression of three individual campgrounds rather than one oversize tent dealership. Loop A houses campsites 1 through 36 on a slight slope. A mix of pines, sweetgum, cedar, and understory trees such as dogwood shades the camps.

Loop B, featuring woodsy sites 37 through 68, is the most isolated and the most popular. It is located on a spur ridge with land dropping off on the outside of the loop, creating a mountain atmosphere. Where the slope is excessive, the sites have been leveled. Try to get one of the sites on the outside of the loop, as these offer more space. Also, the sites are a bit closer together than those on Loop A. Some have parking spurs that pull directly to the sites, while others necessitate a short walk to the camping area. The end of the loop backs against a narrow hollow, creating additional sloping.

Loop C was my choice, with sites 69 through 106. This loop is the most level, has sites that are more widespread than those in Loops A and B, and is the only

RATINGS

Beauty: ✿ ✿ ✿ ✿
Privacy: ✿ ✿ ✿
Spaciousness: ✿ ✿ ✿ ✿
Quiet: ✿ ✿ ✿ ✿
Security: ✿ ✿ ✿ ✿ ✿
Cleanliness: ✿ ✿ ✿ ✿

loop open in winter. This loop is bisected by a cross-road. Some sites along it are open and grassy—perfect in colder months—while pines shade others. Younger hardwoods shade yet other sites. A campground host is here for your safety and convenience, except in winter. Morrow Mountain fills on holiday weekends and a few ideal-weather weekends during spring and fall.

When asked why campers come here, one park ranger summed it up in one word: "Variety." The park offers both waterfront and mountaintop attractions. Lake Tillery, a 17-mile impoundment of the upper Pee Dee River, offers the water recreation. Campers with boats can use the park ramp to ply the lake, fishing for striped bass, largemouth bass, crappie, bream, and catfish. If you don't have a boat, you can rent a canoe or rowboat for exploring the lake. Otherwise, use the 120-foot fishing pier. The park also has the only swimming pool in the North Carolina state park system. Open during the summer, it features a bathhouse constructed of native stone in the 1930s.

The park's trail system stretches from one end of its boundaries to the other. Half the trails are hiker only, while the other half are hiker-and-horse paths. The Rocks Trail leads directly from the campground to an outcrop overlooking Lake Tillery. The Hattaway Mountain Trail is less used and more challenging, offering winter vistas. Take the Sugarloaf Mountain Trail and the Morrow Mountain Trail for far-reaching views of the lake and land beyond. Of course, a road leads to instant vistas atop Morrow Mountain. Speaking of roads, bicyclers like to pedal their way around the park; be advised, though, that some of these roads are steep.

Visitors should explore the park's history, too. The Kron House re-creates the home of the area's first doctor, Francis Kron. The home, office, infirmary, and greenhouse appear much as they did in the 1870s. Weekend interpretive programs tell of the events of Kron's day and other aspects of the state park. You ought to take the good doctor's advice and settle down here for a spell. Oh, and bring your tent.

KEY INFORMATION

ADDRESS:	49104 Morrow Mountain Rd. Albemarle, NC 28001
OPERATED BY:	North Carolina State Parks
INFORMATION:	(704) 982-4402; ncparks.gov; reservations: (877) 722-6762
OPEN:	Year-round; only C Loop open in winter
SITES:	106
EACH SITE:	Picnic table, fire grate, lantern post, tent pad
ASSIGNMENT:	First come, first served and by reservation
REGISTRATION:	Ranger will come by to register you
FACILITIES:	Hot showers, flush toilets, water spigots
PARKING:	At campsites only
FEE:	$15
ELEVATION:	450 feet
RESTRICTIONS:	*Pets:* On leash only *Fires:* In fire rings only *Alcohol:* Prohibited *Vehicles:* On designated parking pad *Other:* 14-day stay limit in 30-day period

MAP

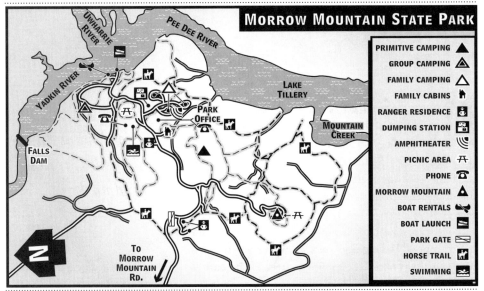

MORROW MOUNTAIN STATE PARK

PRIMITIVE CAMPING	▲
GROUP CAMPING	◬
FAMILY CAMPING	△
FAMILY CABINS	🏠
RANGER RESIDENCE	🏠
DUMPING STATION	🚽
AMPHITHEATER	《
PICNIC AREA	⛱
PHONE	☎
MORROW MOUNTAIN	▲
BOAT RENTALS	🛶
BOAT LAUNCH	🚤
PARK GATE	✕
HORSE TRAIL	🏇
SWIMMING	🏊

GETTING THERE

From downtown Badin, take Falls Road 0.1 mile to Boyden Street. Turn right on Boyden Street, staying left past the golf course and traveling 2.4 miles to Morrow Mountain Road. Turn left on Morrow Mountain Road, and follow it 1.5 miles to reach the park.

GPS COORDINATES

UTM Zone (WGS84) 17S
Easting 0584630
Northing 3914400
Latitude 35 22' 17.9"
Longitude 80 4' 6.4"

25
PILOT MOUNTAIN STATE PARK

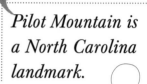

NORTH CAROLINA has many special mountains, but when it comes to memorable and distinct landmarks, Pilot Mountain takes the cake. On the edge of the Piedmont, the mountain—named for its status as a way marker for all who passed through the area—rises from the surrounding lands to climax in a circular peak of nearly vertical rock walls with a wooded cap. The park is now a great destination for tent campers. Hiking and rock climbing are the primary pastimes here. The mountain area of the park is complemented by an additional segment on the Yadkin River that has a living history farm, fishing and canoeing opportunities, and hiking trails.

The campground is situated, not surprisingly, on a slope of Pilot Mountain. Before you imagine having to buckle yourself in to keep from rolling off a hill, realize that the sites have been leveled, for the most part, and all sites have level tent pads, making mountainside slumber more likely.

The paved campground loop has paved parking spurs to minimize erosion and keep your car from sliding off the mountain. Overhead, chestnut oaks, dogwoods, and hickories shade the campsites. Mountain laurels and young trees make a passable understory. Many of the sites are separated from the parking spur, necessitating a short walk into the woods and sometimes up or down steps. This short walk actually increases campsite privacy, but squeezing in sites where the terrain allows compromises their size. Most sites are average in size, while others are small. Limiting your gear will increase your site choices. Cruise around the loop, passing the Grindstone Trail beyond site 16. A modern bathhouse stands near site 25. From here, the loop circles downhill. Sometimes, a site's picnic table and tent pad are spaced a bit apart because of the terrain. However, the sloping mountainside enhances the

> *Pilot Mountain is a North Carolina landmark.*

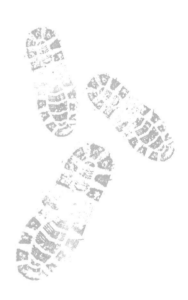

RATINGS

Beauty: ✩ ✩ ✩ ✩
Privacy: ✩ ✩ ✩
Spaciousness: ✩ ✩
Quiet: ✩ ✩ ✩ ✩
Security: ✩ ✩ ✩ ✩ ✩
Cleanliness: ✩ ✩ ✩

ADDRESS:	1792 Pilot Knob Park Rd. Pinnacle, NC 27699
OPERATED BY:	North Carolina State Parks
INFORMATION:	(336) 325-2355; ncparks.gov; reservations: (877) 722-6762
OPEN:	March 15–November 30
SITES:	49
EACH SITE:	Picnic table, fire ring, tent pad
ASSIGNMENT:	First come, first served and by reservation
REGISTRATION:	Ranger will come by to register you
FACILITIES:	Hot showers, flush toilets, water spigots
PARKING:	At campsites only
FEE:	$12
ELEVATION:	1,000 feet
RESTRICTIONS:	*Pets:* On leash only *Fires:* In fire rings only *Alcohol:* Prohibited *Vehicles:* 32-foot trailer-length limit *Other:* 14-day stay limit in 30-day period

camping atmosphere here on Pilot Mountain, where 95 percent of the sites are desirable.

Weekdays are very quiet, and, surprisingly, Pilot Mountain fills only on holiday weekends. Any other time you should be able to get a site. You will be sharing the campground with young couples, families, the occasional rock climber, and other folks who come here to get a firsthand look at the unusual mountain.

The view looking up at Pilot Mountain as you arrive arouses a curiosity to see what it's like looking down on the surrounding landscape. Here are the statistics: Pilot Mountain stands 2,421 feet high, more than 1,400 feet above the surrounding countryside. On a clear day, you can see more than 3,000 square miles from Little Pinnacle Overlook.

More than 27 miles of trails course through the park's mountain and river sections. Take the Ledge Spring Trail for a trip along sheer rock bluffs. The Jomeokee Trail circles the crest of the circular mountain. The Grindstone Trail leads from the campground and allows access to the other high-country paths. The longest trail is the Corridor Trail, which connects the river and mountain sections of the park. The river section of the park is centered on the Yadkin Islands, on the Yadkin River. The Horne Creek Trail starts near the Horne Creek Living Historical Farm where, on weekends, folks dressed in early-20th-century period clothes go about the business of farm life from that era. Check ahead with the park to make sure a demonstration is going on during your visit. The nearby Yadkin River offers 165 miles of canoeing possibilities. The Shoals Access site is just upstream of the Yadkin Islands. Your river experience should contrast well with your more-solid explorations from atop Pilot Mountain.

MAP

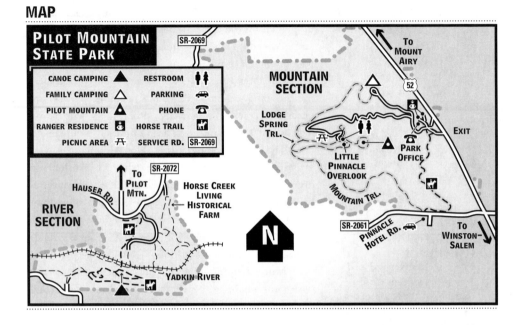

GETTING THERE

From Winston-Salem, drive north on US 52 and take the Pilot Mountain exit, which is not numbered. (This is the next exit after Exit 129 for the town of Pinnacle.) Turn left on Pilot Mountain Road, and follow it 1 mile to the park, on your left.

GPS COORDINATES

UTM Zone (WGS84) 17S
Easting 0546590
Northing 1099010
Latitude 30 20' 37.3"
Longitude 80 28' 50.2"

> *This off-the-beaten-path campground offers access to the lesser-used Uwharrie Trail.*

MY EXPECTATIONS were low before arriving at West Morris Mountain Campground. Most of the smaller recreation destinations of the Uwharrie National Forest had been broken-down hunt camps. I was hoping against hope for something good, and my hopes were realized on this ridgetop. The campground was in great shape. And the master path of this national forest, Uwharrie Trail, is less than a mile away from the campground. Furthermore, a side trail connects West Morris Mountain to Uwharrie Trail.

The mountains of the Uwharrie are not like those of western North Carolina, but they do offer distinct topographical relief, a milder climate, and much easier access from the Piedmont than the Appalachians to the west. Elevations generally range from 400 to 900 feet, and the crowd numbers are much lower here as well. Although lacking the height of other North Carolina mountains, this area has its beauty.

My fall tour of the Uwharries was well timed. The yellow sugar maples and red dogwoods were bursting with color, contrasting with a cobalt-blue sky. That nip in the air offered brisk relief from the long, hot summer.

The campground is set on the western shoulder of Morris Mountain. Pass a few sites with tent pads in a mix of grass and woods before entering the main campground. The main campground is strung out on a classic loop. The sites have been rehabilitated and are in good shape. A hardwood forest of maples, oaks, and dogwoods with assorted pines shades the sites; heavy vegetation screens them from one another. Site 1 is on the loop's inside. Site 2 offers privacy. Site 3 is away from the loop. Site 5 is next to a modern vault toilet. Sites 6 and 7 are heavily shaded. Site 8 is larger than most. Sites 9 and 10 are on the outside of the loop and overlook a hollow. Sites 11, 12, and 13 will suit most campers. Site 14 is a handicapped site. A second vault

RATINGS

Beauty: ☆ ☆ ☆ ☆
Privacy: ☆ ☆ ☆ ☆ ☆
Spaciousness: ☆ ☆ ☆
Quiet: ☆ ☆ ☆ ☆
Security: ☆ ☆
Cleanliness: ☆ ☆ ☆

toilet is near here. Bring your own drinking water.

The sites are well spaced from one another but are small to average in size, which is good for tent campers since it discourages bigger rigs. Realistically, West Morris Mountain is too primitive for the non–tent-camping set. This campground never fills.

Expect to create your own adventures here. The Morris Mountain Trail lies near the loop's beginning. Pass around a metal gate, and begin climbing to reach Uwharrie Trail after 0.75 miles. Here Uwharrie Trail leaves right and continues forward on the old roadbed. Joe Moffitt, who grew up in the Uwharrie Mountains, built the 21-mile trail. It passes over ridges, into stream-beds, and by old homesites and cemeteries. Unfortunately, loops are not possible at the northern end of the forest near West Morris Mountain. However, the 9.5-mile Dutchman's Creek Trail loops with Uwharrie Trail in the south end of the forest.

The Birkhead Mountains Wilderness is not far from West Morris Mountain. This 5,000-acre preserve has stands of old-growth hardwoods broken by clear streams. Parts of it were settled, and you can still see remnants of homesites and even gold-mining operations. The wilderness trailhead can be reached by turning right out of the campground and staying on Ophir Road as it becomes Burney Mill Road, where you cross into Randolph County. Continue on to the intersection of Lassiter Mill Road, and turn right. Keep north on Lassiter Mill Road and look for the trailhead on your right. Once here, hike Robbins Branch, Birkhead, and Hannah's Branch trails to make a stellar 6.9-mile loop. A wilderness map is available from the ranger station in Troy, as is a Uwharrie Trail map. Order both forest maps, and then discover the lesser-known Uwharrie Mountains.

KEY INFORMATION

ADDRESS:	789 NC 24/27 East Troy, NC 27371
OPERATED BY:	U.S. Forest Service
INFORMATION:	(910) 576-6391; cs.unca.edu/nfsnc
OPEN:	Year-round
SITES:	17
EACH SITE:	Picnic table, fire grate, lantern post, tent pad
ASSIGNMENT:	First come, first served; no reservations
REGISTRATION:	Self-registration on site
FACILITIES:	Vault toilet
PARKING:	At campsites only
FEE:	$10
ELEVATION:	450 feet
RESTRICTIONS:	*Pets:* On leash only *Fires:* In fire rings only *Alcohol:* Prohibited *Vehicles:* None *Other:* No trash cans—pack it in, pack it out

MAP

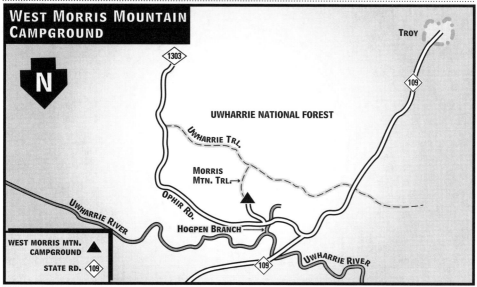

GETTING THERE

From Troy, head north on NC 109 9 miles to Ophir Road, NC 1303. Turn right on Ophir Road, and follow it 1 mile to the campground, on your right.

GPS COORDINATES

UTM Zone (WGS84) 17S
Easting 0590900
Northing 3919820
Latitude 35 25' 8.8"
Longitude 79 59' 52.1"

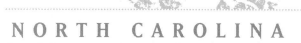

NORTH CAROLINA
COAST AND **COASTAL PLAIN**

27
CAROLINA BEACH STATE PARK

THIS AREA OF THE CAROLINAS certainly has some amazing natural attributes, but the most unusual of all may be the Venus flytrap. Perhaps you have heard of it. The modified leaves of this plant close rapidly when an insect touches tiny hairs on the leaves' inside, trapping the insect, which then becomes dinner. The Venus flytrap grows only on land located within a 60-mile radius of Wilmington, North Carolina. Carolina Beach State Park has a trail where you can see this unusual plant. The park also has a fine, lesser-used campground as well as many attractions within a 10-mile radius of the campground, such as beaches, historic sites, and even an aquarium.

With all there is to do here, you should find the campground very appealing as a base camp. It is located in piney woods near Snow's Cut, a waterway connecting the wide Cape Fear River to the Intracoastal Waterway. Pine trees tower over the two campground loops. Live oaks, water oaks, and other hardwoods are mixed in with the pines. Clumpy brush grows here and there among the woods, adding privacy. A drive on the paved campground road through the first loop reveals large sites with sand-and-pine-needle floors. The Snow's Cut Trail leads toward a maritime forest near campsite 21. We enjoyed site 25, where the filtering sunlight helped dry our gear after a storm pushed through the previous night. A bathhouse centers the loop.

A short road with large campsites along it leads to the second loop, which hosts sites 48 through 82 and opens only when the first loop fills. The sites look little used in this loop, but the first loop doesn't get a whole lot of business either. The second loop, from which the Sugarloaf Trail leaves at site 54, also has large camps and a bathhouse in the center.

This campground has an unusual system for claiming campsites. A little green tag hangs below each

> *Many attractions are within a short drive of this lesser-used oceanside campground.*

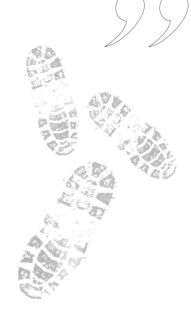

RATINGS

Beauty: ✪ ✪ ✪ ✪
Privacy: ✪ ✪ ✪
Spaciousness: ✪ ✪ ✪ ✪
Quiet: ✪ ✪ ✪
Security: ✪ ✪ ✪ ✪ ✪
Cleanliness: ✪ ✪ ✪

ADDRESS: P.O. Box 475
Carolina Beach,
NC 28428

OPERATED BY: North Carolina
State Parks

INFORMATION: (910) 458-8206;
ncparks.gov;
reservations:
(877) 722-6762

OPEN: Year-round

SITES: 83

EACH SITE: Picnic table,
fire ring

ASSIGNMENT: First come,
first served and
by reservation

REGISTRATION: At park store and
marina

FACILITIES: Hot showers,
flush toilets,
water spigots

PARKING: At campsites only

FEE: $15

ELEVATION: 10 feet

RESTRICTIONS: *Pets:* On leash only
Fires: In fire rings
only
Alcohol: Prohibited
Vehicles: No more
than two per site
Other: No more
than six campers
per site

unoccupied and numbered site post. When you find a site you like, grab the green tag, take it to the park store and marina, and register there. The campground fills most weekends from Memorial Day through Fourth of July weekend. After that, the heat keeps most campers away until fall, when cooler-weather weekends become busy but usually do not see the campground full. A campsite can be had most spring weekends and any-time during winter. We came during fall—the weather was ideal, and the insects weren't bothersome.

There are beach accesses aplenty near Carolina Beach State Park on nearby Pleasure Island. I recom-mend driving 5 miles to Fort Fisher State Recreation Area. It features 7 miles of state-owned beach with summer lifeguards in the designated ocean-swimming area. Four-wheel-drive vehicles can access other areas along the beach. The recreation area is popular with beachcombers. The North Carolina Aquarium at Fort Fisher is a great place to check out marine life up close, and Fort Fisher State Historic Site, where you can learn about the history of this Confederate Civil War bunker, is located nearby. Many folks like to tour the USS *North Carolina* battleship, conspicuously located in the Cape Fear River near Wilmington.

Don't forget, though, about all the fun stuff to do at Carolina Beach State Park. The area is laced with hiking trails that crisscross numerous natural communi-ties. The Flytrap Trail features the famous Venus fly-trap. The Sugarloaf Trail passes through tidal flats and pinewoods. Snow's Cut Trail leads to the Intracoastal Waterway. The 6-plus miles of trails are hiked mostly during cooler months.

For anglers, a fishing deck leading into the Cape Fear River is near the park marina. This location attracts fishermen going for croaker, flounder, and striped bass, in all types of weather. The marina sells plenty of bait and tackle, and campers with boats will enjoy the con-venience of the boat launch.

With an abundance of recreational and sightsee-ing opportunities close by, camping at Carolina Beach is pleasurable as well as convenient.

MAP

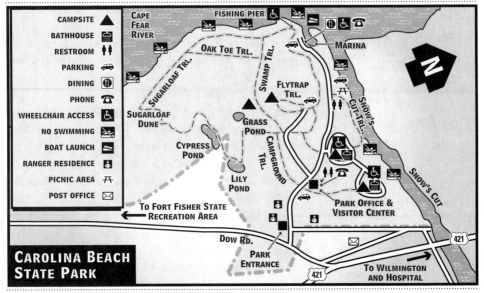

CAMPSITE ▲
BATHHOUSE
RESTROOM
PARKING
DINING
PHONE ☎
WHEELCHAIR ACCESS ♿
NO SWIMMING
BOAT LAUNCH
RANGER RESIDENCE
PICNIC AREA 🛆
POST OFFICE ✉

CAPE FEAR RIVER
FISHING PIER
MARINA
OAK TOE TRL.
SUGARLOAF TRL.
SWAMP TRL.
FLYTRAP TRL.
SUGARLOAF DUNE
GRASS POND
SNOW'S CUT TRL.
CYPRESS POND
CAMPGROUND TRL.
LILY POND
SNOW'S CUT
PARK OFFICE & VISITOR CENTER
To FORT FISHER STATE RECREATION AREA
DOW RD.
PARK ENTRANCE
421
To WILMINGTON AND HOSPITAL

CAROLINA BEACH STATE PARK

GETTING THERE

From Wilmington, drive south on US 421 15 miles, crossing the Intracoastal Waterway. Turn right on Dow Road past the Intracoastal Waterway, shortly reaching the park, on your right.

GPS COORDINATES

UTM Zone (WGS84) 18S
Easting 0231600
Northing 3771290
Latitude 34 2' 59"
Longitude 77 54' 27.9"

> *This underutilized campground stands next to some surprising terrain on the coastal plain.*

OFTEN STATE PARKS are established to protect a natural resource unique to the state. Cliffs of the Neuse fits this mold. Hills are limited here on the coastal plain, and cliffs are rare. Interesting geologic events occurred to form the cliffs along the Neuse River. In 1944, local landowner Lionel Weil proposed that this unusual area, which also harbors a mixture of plants representing different areas of the state, be preserved as a state park. Private individuals banded together to donate the land for the park to the state of North Carolina. More property was added later and an infrastructure built to complement the cliffs, including a lake, trails, and an uncrowded campground that is a great weekend retreat.

The campground lies beneath rich woodland on slightly sloping land. Tall pines mix with a variety of hardwoods, including hickory, beech, and water oak. The brushy understory of holly, young sweetgum, and other small trees can be thick in one spot and open in another, creating privacy at one campsite and openness at the next. The first few sites are wooded around the edges and open in the center. Pine needles and sand carpet the sites. I enjoyed site 12 because it shaded a strong September sun. Luckily, a cool night followed. Barefoot campers should avoid site 14, as a holly tree stands in its center.

The loop curves around and reaches an area with limited shade starting at campsite 20. Thick brush shields the sites on their sides, but they are open overhead. Lush grass carpets these sites, which show less use than the shaded ones. Thick woods resume past site 25. The loop curves uphill, making the last few sites a bit too sloped for good camping.

Overall, the sites are large and desirable for tent campers, making the light use of this campground surprising. It only fills on holiday weekends, so Cliffs of the

RATINGS

Beauty: ☆ ☆ ☆
Privacy: ☆ ☆ ☆
Spaciousness: ☆ ☆ ☆ ☆
Quiet: ☆ ☆ ☆ ☆
Security: ☆ ☆ ☆ ☆ ☆
Cleanliness: ☆ ☆ ☆

Neuse is great for avoiding the crowds at other times, especially during spring and fall. Ideal-weather weekends during these seasons only fill half the 35 sites.

Water spigots are laid out at convenient intervals along the loop; the bathhouse is accessed by trails spoking into the loop's center. For your safety, the park gates are locked every night. If an emergency occurs, use the number posted at the park office near the campground. Rangers live on site and can assist you.

An emergency may be the only time you have to get in your car while at the park. Access to all facilities is just a walk away. For example, a trail leads from the campground to the park museum. Here, the formation of the Cliffs of the Neuse is explained in a manner that even the geologically challenged like me can understand; park history is detailed as well. The actual Cliffs of the Neuse stand just feet from the museum. Walk along the split-rail fence to garner some views that are unusual for this region, while the Neuse River beckons below. Take the 350 Yard Trail along the cliff to the river's edge. Here, anglers may be lazing away the day, going for largemouth bass but more likely catching bream and bluegill. The trail bridges gurgling Mill Creek, where a facility for grinding corn once stood. The Galax Trail starts across the water. Here lies an isolated pocket of the galax plant, normally a mountain species of ground cover. The Bird Trail loops along the Neuse River, providing more bank-fishing opportunities there as well as along Still Creek, where whiskey was once made. These trails are great for families with kids or folks who just want a light leg-stretcher.

Seeing the Neuse River made me want to go on a float trip. Conveniently, a shuttle and canoe-livery service is located on the Neuse River near the park. The most popular run is from the NC 111 bridge down to the hamlet of Seven Springs, a distance of 8 miles. For more information, contact Tony Daw at (919) 734-2291.

The state park offers water recreation of its own. The upper reaches of Mill Creek have been dammed, forming a spring-fed, 11-acre lake. There is an elaborate swim area, with a wide swim beach adjacent to a large, grassy lawn. A changing building and snack bar are also located here. The swim area has recently been

KEY INFORMATION

ADDRESS: 345-A Park Entrance Rd. Seven Springs, NC 28578

OPERATED BY: North Carolina State Parks

INFORMATION: (919) 778-6234; ncparks.gov; reservations: (877) 722-6762

OPEN: March 15– November 30

SITES: 35

EACH SITE: Picnic table, fire grate

ASSIGNMENT: First come, first served and by reservation

REGISTRATION: Ranger will come by to register you

FACILITIES: Hot showers, flush toilets, water spigots

PARKING: At campsites only

FEE: $15

ELEVATION: 125 feet

RESTRICTIONS: *Pets:* On leash only
Fires: In fire rings only
Alcohol: Prohibited
Vehicles: No more than two per site
Other: 14-day stay limit in a 30-day period

MAP

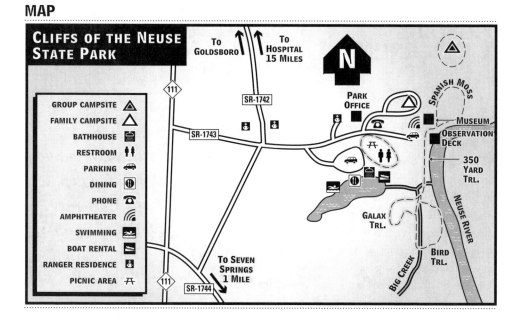

CLIFFS OF THE NEUSE STATE PARK

To GOLDSBORO
To HOSPITAL 15 MILES

N

111

SR-1742

SR-1743

PARK OFFICE

SPANISH MOSS

MUSEUM

OBSERVATION DECK

350 YARD TRL.

GROUP CAMPSITE	△
FAMILY CAMPSITE	△
BATHHOUSE	🛁
RESTROOM	🚻
PARKING	🚗
DINING	🍴
PHONE	☎
AMPHITHEATER	🎦
SWIMMING	🏊
BOAT RENTAL	⛵
RANGER RESIDENCE	🏠
PICNIC AREA	🏕

GALAX TRL.

NEUSE RIVER

BIG CREEK

BIRD TRL.

To SEVEN SPRINGS 1 MILE

111

SR-1744

GETTING THERE

From Goldsboro, drive east on US 70 5 miles to NC 111. Turn right on NC 111, and follow it 9 miles to Park Entrance Road (SR 1743). Turn left on Park Entrance Road, and follow it into the park.

renovated, so it's even better than before. As you have read, the unique features that are the Cliffs of the Neuse have been protected and enhanced by this state park. Now come check them out for yourself.

GPS COORDINATES

UTM Zone (WGS84) 18S
Easting 0237150
Northing 3903120
Latitude 35 14' 18.9"
Longitude 77 53' 17.8"

29
FRISCO
CAMPGROUND

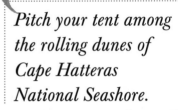

FRISCO CAMPGROUND offers some phenomenal oceanside scenery. Located in the Cape Hatteras National Seashore, the campground is situated among dunes so hilly that you might think you were in the mountains instead of at the beach. OK, that's an exaggeration, but oceanside topography doesn't get much more vertical than this in the Tar Heel State. Beach activities such as surf fishing, beachcombing, kayaking, and visiting lighthouses are on the agenda. Or maybe the agenda is to just sit by the Atlantic Ocean and listen to the waves roll in.

Pitch your tent among the rolling dunes of Cape Hatteras National Seashore.

But make no mistake—this oceanside environment is harsh and unforgiving. This is what accounts for the stark beauty of the Outer Banks: a relentless ocean pounding against the sand, rolling dunes where sea oats cling to life, wind-sculpted trees growing in dune swales, a strong sun beating down on the very openness that is the banks. The campground reflects this stark beauty. The sites are appealing, but they are exposed to wind, sun, and mosquitoes.

The campground is laid out in a big loop with six roads crossing it. The loop overlays a series of dunes that are ever increasing in height as you head away from the ocean, which runs parallel to the campground and is about 150 yards distant. Scattered cedars, oaks, and pines grow mostly brushy, looking nothing like they would on the mainland. The wind keeps these trees from growing straight and tall. They are most stunted on the tops of the dunes, if they grow there at all. In the swales, where the wind is not as strong, the trees more resemble their inland cousins, but trees that grow over a person's head are few. Nevertheless, campsites with even a modicum of shade will be snapped up. Most sites are completely in the open, cutting privacy to a minimum.

As the main loop curves around, pass some pine

RATINGS

Beauty: ✿ ✿ ✿ ✿ ✿
Privacy: ✿
Spaciousness: ✿ ✿
Quiet: ✿ ✿ ✿ ✿
Security: ✿ ✿ ✿ ✿ ✿
Cleanliness: ✿ ✿

ADDRESS: 53415 Billy Mitchell Rd. Frisco, NC 27936

OPERATED BY: National Park Service

INFORMATION: (252) 473-2111; nps.gov/caha

OPEN: Friday of Easter weekend–mid-October

SITES: 127

EACH SITE: Picnic table, upright grill

ASSIGNMENT: First come, first served; no reservations

REGISTRATION: At campground entrance booth

FACILITIES: Cold showers, water spigots, flush toilets

PARKING: At campsites only

FEE: $20

ELEVATION: 50 feet

RESTRICTIONS: *Pets:* On leash only *Fires:* In upright grills only, below high tide line on beach *Alcohol:* At campsites only *Vehicles:* No more than two per site; must be parked on paved surface

trees in the low area between the campground and the beach, which is accessed by two boardwalks. The road rises remarkably high, maybe a couple hundred feet. The sites on the back of the loop begin to overlook the ocean, offering stunning panoramas. Just like any sites here, these have their pluses and minuses. The open sites will have the wind, which cuts down on mosquitoes, but if the wind is cold, then the openness is a negative. If the sun is blaring down, as it often is, then the lack of shade can be a problem. Bringing a screen shelter can eliminate both sun and bug problems. Many sites are small, so you will have to be flexible in how you set up camp. I stayed in site P-56 and enjoyed the afternoon shade, but the mosquitoes were a bit troublesome.

Campers usually end up finding a site to suit them (do some driving around once you get here). No matter your location, a bathhouse and water spigot are close by. Frisco fills on major holidays and a few other perfect-weather weekends in summer. Otherwise, you should be able to get a site.

Four-wheel-drive vehicles can access the beach at many areas of Cape Hatteras National Seashore. These access points are referred to as ramps, one of which is adjacent to the campground. Most campers just use the boardwalks to reach the beach by foot. In either case, you have miles of shoreline to enjoy, whether you are surf casting or surfing with a board. A fishing pier is just west of the campground, as is a designated swim beach with a bathhouse.

Cape Hatteras Lighthouse is just a short drive away. It made the news some years ago when it was moved to keep it from falling into the shifting sea. You can climb the lighthouse and get a grand view, or you can walk the nearby Buxton Woods Trail, operated in conjunction with the Nature Conservancy. Supplies are available in the village of Frisco, which is conveniently just a mile from the campground. And after staying a night or two, a mile may be all you will want to get away from here.

MAP

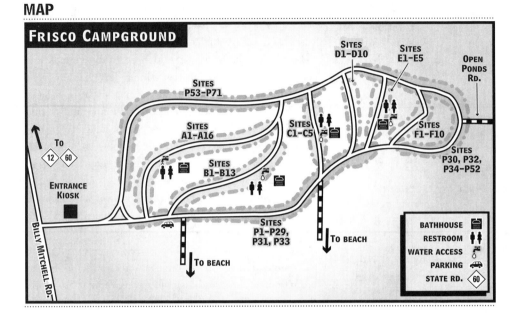

FRISCO CAMPGROUND

SITES D1–D10

SITES E1–E5

OPEN PONDS RD.

SITES P53–P71

SITES A1–A16

SITES C1–C5

SITES F1–F10

To 12 60

SITES B1–B13

SITES P30, P32, P34–P52

ENTRANCE KIOSK

SITES P1–P29, P31, P33

To BEACH

To BEACH

BILLY MITCHELL RD.

BATHHOUSE	
RESTROOM	
WATER ACCESS	
PARKING	
STATE RD.	60

GETTING THERE

From the intersection of US 64/264 and US 158 just south of Nags Head, drive south on NC 12 60 miles to the hamlet of Frisco. Turn left on Billy Mitchell Road, and follow it 1 mile to reach the campground.

GPS COORDINATES

UTM Zone (WGS84) 18S

Easting 0450850

Northing 3899100

Latitude 35 12' 38.8"

Longitude 75 33' 17.2"

> *"Enjoy some of the coastal plain's finest wetlands at this quiet state park."*

THIS STATE PARK has a fine environmental-education center that offers first-rate displays and information about North Carolina's wet-lands, where the interplay between land, river, and ocean forms a rich ecosystem that is explained for all to understand. The center is worth a stop, but an even better idea is to explore this state park's ecosystem for yourself. Gain firsthand knowledge about the preserve on the edge of the Pamlico River via foot and pad-dling trails, or launch your activities from the park campground, which could hardly get better from this tent camper's point of view.

The so-called primitive campground is set on a piece of high ground between Flatty and Goose creeks. A narrow gravel road stretches out beneath tall loblolly pines, complemented by hickory, oak, holly, and bay trees. The forest understory is light. Be careful driving the campground road, as trees grow so close alongside it that you might nick one with your car. A sign at the beginning of the campground states "No large RVs." Soon come to campsite 1. A gravel parking spur leads to a large site shaded by pines, oaks, and hollies. Just like the other sites, one part of the site is sand for plac-ing your tent. Site 1 was so alluring that I claimed it immediately without looking at the rest of the camp-ground, but it's far from the only good site here. Site 2 is a good 75 yards down the road—the sites here are as widespread as you are going to get—and has a gravel parking pad with a short walkway leading to the site. (Most sites here require a short walk to reach the actual camping areas.) Past one of four water spigots, site 3 is a double, 200 feet from the road. Site 4 is a drive-up site. Across from site 4 is one of two composting toilets using the latest ventilation technology, which does make a difference in the odor department.

Keep going down the road. Site 5 is also a drive-up

RATINGS

Beauty: ✿ ✿ ✿ ✿
Privacy: ✿ ✿ ✿ ✿ ✿
Spaciousness: ✿ ✿ ✿ ✿ ✿
Quiet: ✿ ✿ ✿ ✿ ✿
Security: ✿ ✿ ✿ ✿ ✿
Cleanliness: ✿ ✿ ✿ ✿ ✿

site and has an upright grill in addition to a fire ring. Site 6 is a walk-in site in a shady flat. (All the sites here are level, by the way, and designated parking spots are provided for each walk-in site.) Site 7 is on the right, across the road from Flatty Creek Trail. Site 8 is a walk-in site scattered with pines. Site 9 is another walk-in site. Site 10 has many hardwoods shading it. The last two sites, 11 and 12, require a longer walk but are also closest to Goose Creek. Site 12 looks toward water on three sides, though the water is a good 100 feet away. An auto turnaround is at the end of the road, along with an observation deck that stretches into Goose Creek.

Spring and fall are the best times to camp at Goose Creek. The campground fills a couple of great-weather weekends per season. A site will be available any time of the year during the week, although summer is too hot and buggy.

Now, explore the wetlands that make Goose Creek so special. You may want to visit the environmental education center first to gain an understanding of the ecosystem and to learn what to look for, then take off. The Palmetto Boardwalk behind the nature center offers interpretive signage showing you the wetlands firsthand. Campers can use the small, sandy shore at the campground's edge to launch their canoes or kayaks into the water. Here, you can join the Goose Creek Canoe Trail, which explores not only the natural history of the area but also the human history. Check out relics of an old logging operation in addition to wildflowers and wildlife, especially birds. Flatty and Mallard creeks are also good paddling destinations, as is the shoreline along Pamlico River. The brackish river supports both saltwater and freshwater species, so bring your pole and angle for flounder, bream, black drum, and largemouth bass. A swim beach, which requires a short walk, is on the Pamlico, too.

Landlubbers have choices as well. Ivey Gut Trail leaves from the upper end of the campground and curves alongside Goose Creek for a 2-mile, one-way trek. Flatty Creek Trail is also accessible directly from the campground. It makes a 1-mile loop through the woods and across boardwalks to reach an observation deck along Flatty Creek. Goose Creek Trail is the

ADDRESS:	2190 Camp Leach Rd. Washington, NC 27889
OPERATED BY:	North Carolina State Parks
INFORMATION:	(252) 923-0052; ncparks.gov; reservations: (877) 722-6762
OPEN:	Year-round
SITES:	12
EACH SITE:	Picnic table, fire ring, lantern post
ASSIGNMENT:	First come, first served and by reservation
REGISTRATION:	Ranger will come by to register you
FACILITIES:	Water spigot, vault toilet
PARKING:	At campsites only
FEE:	$9
ELEVATION:	10 feet
RESTRICTIONS:	*Pets:* On leash only *Fires:* In fire rings only *Alcohol:* Prohibited *Vehicles:* None *Other:* 14-day stay limit in 30-day period

MAP

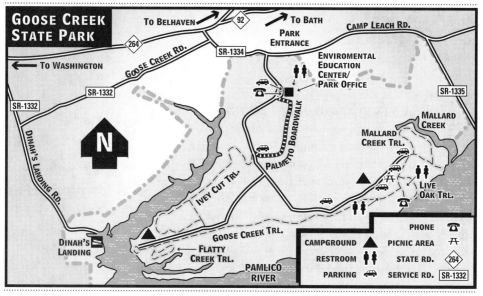

GETTING THERE

From Washington, head east on US 264 9 miles to Camp Leach Road (SR 1334). Turn right on Camp Leach Road, and follow it 2.2 miles to the park.

park's longest, at 2.9 miles. Here, you can enjoy some of the park's three types of primary wetlands—hardwood swamp, cypress gum swamp, and brackish marsh. Ragged Point Trail leads to a boardwalk and observation deck. Live Oak Trail travels beneath stately trees draped with Spanish moss. Exploring this park is a joy you can experience many times over, especially with such a nice campground.

GPS COORDINATES

UTM Zone (WGS84) 18S
Easting 0324940
Northing 3927210
Latitude 35 28' 29.6"
Longitude 76 55' 44.4"

31
JONES LAKE
STATE PARK

HAVE YOU EVER HEARD OF BAY LAKES? These natural wonders stretch from Florida to New Jersey but are most prominent in the Carolinas. They are usually oval shaped, pointed on a northwest-to-southeast axis, and no deeper than 10 feet. Theories about the origins of these lakes range from meteors crashing into Earth to gigantic prehistoric whales carving holes in ancient shallow seas with their tails. *Bay* refers to the preponderance of sweet bay and red bay trees growing around them. A bay lake called Jones Lake is the centerpiece of this quiet state park with a good campground that is simply not used as much as it deserves.

The campground and recreation areas of Jones Lake State Park are on the southeastern shore of the 224-acre lake, which is ringed by cypress, bay, titi, and other moisture-tolerant flora. The campground is situated in slightly higher, sandier terrain. Here, longleaf pine and turkey oaks predominate. These two trees are part of the longleaf-wiregrass ecosystem, which once covered more than 20 million acres in the Southeast. This open woodland makes for a very attractive campground setting.

A paved road loops around the campground. The large campsites have floors of sand and pine needles. Pond and loblolly pines also grow among the longleafs. Turkey oaks, with their short limbs and scrubby appearance, stand beneath the pines. Young bay trees, sassafras, and cane shoot from the ground. The sites have a mixture of sun and shade, but are more open than not. At virtually any other campground, privacy might be compromised, but this attractive destination's surprising unpopularity will likely leave you with no neighbors around.

Beyond campsite 7, a path leads from the campground to the Lake Trail and a fishing pier. The vegetation thickens as a wetland backs the sites. Pass the

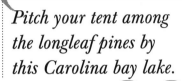

> *Pitch your tent among the longleaf pines by this Carolina bay lake.*

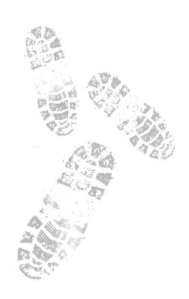

RATINGS

Beauty: ✰ ✰ ✰ ✰
Privacy: ✰ ✰ ✰
Spaciousness: ✰ ✰ ✰ ✰
Quiet: ✰ ✰ ✰ ✰
Security: ✰ ✰ ✰ ✰ ✰
Cleanliness: ✰ ✰ ✰ ✰

ADDRESS: 4117 NC 242 North
Elizabethtown,
NC 28337

OPERATED BY: North Carolina
State Parks

INFORMATION: (910) 588-4550;
ncparks.gov;
reservations:
(877) 722-6762

OPEN: March 15–
November 30

SITES: 20

EACH SITE: Picnic table, fire
grate, trash can

ASSIGNMENT: First come,
first served and
by reservation

REGISTRATION: Ranger will come
by to register you

FACILITIES: Hot showers,
flush toilets,
water spigots

PARKING: At campsites only

FEE: $15, $20 for one
electric site

ELEVATION: 75 feet

RESTRICTIONS: *Pets:* On leash only
Fires: In fire rings
only
Alcohol: Prohibited
Vehicles: None
Other: 14-day stay
limit in a 30-day
period

access road to reach the group campground and sites that are more open, though most have enough shade to make it through a hot day. One site at the park has water and electricity.

A small bathhouse is in the center of the loop. Summer and early fall will find younger families from nearby military bases pitching a tent. Campers can count on getting sites just about any weekend, except for summer-holiday weekends. Even then, though, your chances of getting a site are pretty good.

A visitor center stands near Jones Lake and is the center of activity. Interpretive ranger programs are held on weekends. A pretty picnic area, dotted with scattered trees among lush grass, overlooks the lake, and a dock leads out to a boathouse where canoes and paddleboats can be rented at very reasonable rates. The park swim beach is here, too, marked by buoys that extend far out into the dark waters.

If you want to hike, take the Lake Trail. It extends 3 miles, encircling the scenic body of water. Short side trails lead to the lake's edge and afford good views. Beginning near the nature center, you can take a shorter walk on the Nature Trail, which makes a 1-mile loop.

A boat launch enables those with their own watercraft to access the lake; motors of 10 horsepower and below are allowed. Jones Lake is highly acidic, limiting fishing. However, you can vie for yellow perch, pickerel, catfish, and small sunfish. A fishing pier extends into the lake from near the campground for those without boats. Nearby Salters Lake, also a Carolina bay lake within the park's 2,000-plus acres, is managed as a natural area. Visitors can access it after getting a permit from the ranger station. Carved from the surrounding Bladen Lakes State Forest, Jones Lake State Park is quiet and undeveloped, which, as a tent camper, you will enjoy.

MAP

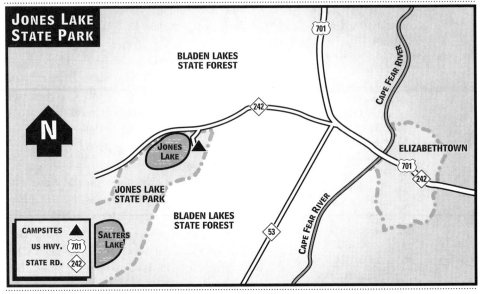

JONES LAKE STATE PARK

BLADEN LAKES
STATE FOREST

N

JONES
LAKE

JONES LAKE
STATE PARK

BLADEN LAKES
STATE FOREST

701

242

53

CAPE FEAR RIVER

CAPE FEAR RIVER

ELIZABETHTOWN

701

242

CAMPSITES
US HWY. 701
STATE RD. 242

SALTERS
LAKE

GETTING THERE

From Elizabethtown,
follow NC 242 north 4 miles
to the state park, which will
be on your left.

GPS COORDINATES

UTM Zone (WGS84) 17S
Easting 0719950
Northing 3839450
Latitude 34 40' 46.3"
Longitude 78 35' 51.5"

"All the camps on the Wild and Scenic Lumber River are walk-in tent sites."

AS A FEDERALLY DESIGNATED Wild and Scenic River, the Lumber is officially special. The state of North Carolina recognizes the river's beauty and added a serpentine state park along it, protecting wild stretches and developing other park units that allow access to riverside camping, as well as water-access points with restrooms and picnic areas. This Princess Ann Unit of the park has a walk-in tent campground where you can enjoy the river and the land around it. Nearby outfitters allow even the boat-less to float down the Lumber and return to this campground, which seems to have tent campers in mind.

The campground is located in lush, dark, and cool woods near the Princess Ann access boat ramp. Seven campsites are grouped together, two of which are directly along the river. The main camping area is set in luxuriant woods on a sloping hill leading toward the Lumber. Water oaks, sweetgums, and understory oaks dominate the forest; smaller bay trees have to work hard to gain light from the thick overhead canopy. A paved path leads to disabled-access campsite 1. This site, like all the others, has been leveled using landscaping timbers. A gravel path continues to site 2. Site 3 is at the lower end of the hill, closer to the river. Site 4 has oaks with outstretched limbs shading it. Site 5 is closer to the river. Site 6 has the farthest walk, but even this is no more than 75 yards. This site is open in the center and has the most privacy of the sites around it. Site 7 is highest on the hill. It is very shady and has pine needles for a carpet, but it's small and was added as an afterthought. A short trail leads to the final two campsites. Walk past the boat ramp and begin heading downstream along the beautiful Lumber. Reach site 8 first, then site 9. Cypress trees draped in Spanish moss stand along the river. A cypress-gum swamp lies on the other side of the campsites. This area is level and shady, exuding the beauty of the river.

RATINGS

Beauty: ✩ ✩ ✩ ✩
Privacy: ✩ ✩ ✩ ✩
Spaciousness: ✩ ✩ ✩
Quiet: ✩ ✩ ✩ ✩
Security: ✩ ✩ ✩ ✩ ✩
Cleanliness: ✩ ✩ ✩ ✩

Bald cypresses, with their knees protruding from the water, line the river, and rich stands of cane overlook the tannin-stained, tea-colored water. A bluff that rises from this side of the river attracted early settlers who formed the community of Princess Ann. Today, the park headquarters, a picnic area, and a hiking trail extend along the bluff, which once served as a buffer against flooding for settlers. A boat ramp is conveniently located beside the camping area. Canoeists and kayakers launch their craft from here for short trips in the immediate area, or they use the ramp as a takeout, making shuttle runs upriver. This dark serpent of flowing watery wilderness runs 115 miles, making overnight wilderness trips viable. Eighty-one of the river miles are designated as Wild and Scenic. If you don't have two cars for a shuttle, River Bend Outfitters, in the nearby town of Fair Bluff, offers shuttle services and rents canoes and kayaks. For more information, call (910) 649-5998. Check the park office for a list of other outfitters operating along the Lumber.

A hiking trail extends from the picnic area along the river and heads upstream for a mile. Check out Griffin's Whorl, where the Lumber reverses its flow before resuming downstream. Along the way, the trail passes an observation deck and fishing pier. Folks angle here for crappie, sunfish, and largemouth bass. Bank fishing also takes places along the shore near the campground. I hope you will take the time to enjoy a tent-camping adventure here on the Lumber River.

KEY INFORMATION

ADDRESS:	2819 Princess Ann Rd. Orrum, NC 28369
OPERATED BY:	North Carolina State Parks
INFORMATION:	(910) 628-9844; ncparks.gov; reservations: (877) 722-6762
OPEN:	Year-round
SITES:	9
EACH SITE:	Picnic table, fire ring, lantern post, tent pad, trash can
ASSIGNMENT:	First come, first served and by reservation
REGISTRATION:	Ranger will come by to register you
FACILITIES:	Water spigot, vault toilet
PARKING:	At boat-ramp parking area
FEE:	$9
ELEVATION:	80 feet
RESTRICTIONS:	*Pets:* On leash only *Fires:* In fire rings only *Alcohol:* Prohibited *Vehicles:* None *Other:* 14-day stay limit in 30-day period

MAP

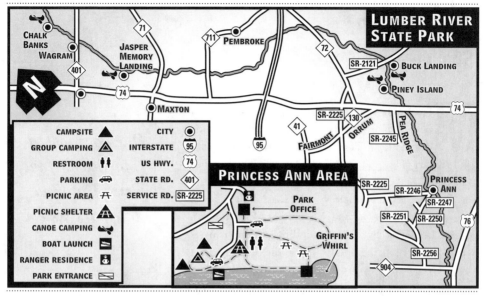

LUMBER RIVER STATE PARK

CHALK BANKS WAGRAM

JASPER MEMORY LANDING

PEMBROKE

BUCK LANDING

PINEY ISLAND

MAXTON

SR-2121

SR-2225

SR-2245

FAIRMONT

ORRUM

PEA RIDGE

PRINCESS ANN

SR-2225

SR-2246

SR-2247

SR-2251

SR-2250

SR-2256

CAMPSITE	▲	CITY	◉
GROUP CAMPING	△	INTERSTATE	95
RESTROOM	♀♂	US HWY.	74
PARKING	🚐	STATE RD.	401
PICNIC AREA	🏕	SERVICE RD.	SR-2225
PICNIC SHELTER	🏕		
CANOE CAMPING	🛶		
BOAT LAUNCH			
RANGER RESIDENCE	🏠		
PARK ENTRANCE	⋈		

PRINCESS ANN AREA

PARK OFFICE

GRIFFIN'S WHIRL

GETTING THERE

From Exit 14 on I-95, take US 74, Andrew Jackson Highway, east 11.3 miles to Creek Road, Service Road 2225 (a sign for Orrum Middle School will be at this turn). Turn right onto Creek Road, and follow it 5.3 miles to Princess Ann Road. Turn left on Princess Ann Road, and follow it 2 miles to reach the Princess Ann Unit of Lumber River State Park, on your left.

GPS COORDINATES

UTM Zone (WGS84) 18S
Easting 0410450
Northing 3880650
Latitude 34 23' 36.9"
Longitude 75 55' 8.7"

MERCHANTS MILLPOND STATE PARK is simply one of North Carolina's finest tent-camping destinations. This quiet getaway in the northeastern part of the state tends to be overlooked because it has neither the glamour of the ocean nor the lure of the mountains; nevertheless, this coastal-plain jewel shines brightly. The actual Merchants Millpond is a mini–Okefenokee Swamp, a brooding wetland ecosystem ideal for canoeing and fishing in the relaxing quiet that only nature can provide. The surrounding high ground has its appeal, too, with many hiking trails traveling the land. To top it off, the campground seems to have been designed for tent campers.

As with all park facilities here, the campground is appealing and well maintained. It is laid out in a classic loop with a mere 20 campsites. Overhead, loblolly pines tower above red and white oaks, maples, and thick understory brush such as myrtle oak. Pine needles carpet the forest floor, and shade is abundant. Elevated tent pads, filled with sand, make staking your tent easy and allow for quick drainage in case of rain. The campsites are located far from one another, which, coupled with the thick woods, makes for maximum privacy. Most sites are on the outside of the loop, but here every site is a winner, no matter where it is located. Small trails lead to the center of the loop, where a modern bathhouse lies. Most sites can accommodate a large tent and screen shelter, if you so desire.

Spring and fall are the best times to visit Merchants Millpond. Summer can be hot and buggy. Late March through April and mid-October are the busiest times, though sites are available just about any weekend. Winter is quiet. Park gates are locked every evening until sunrise, making for maximum safety. An emergency phone is at the ranger station, and a park ranger lives on site.

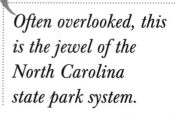

> *Often overlooked, this is the jewel of the North Carolina state park system.*

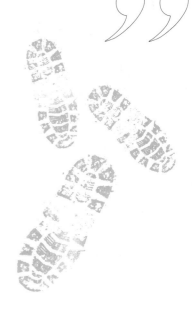

RATINGS

Beauty: ☆ ☆ ☆ ☆ ☆
Privacy: ☆ ☆ ☆ ☆ ☆
Spaciousness: ☆ ☆ ☆ ☆
Quiet: ☆ ☆ ☆ ☆ ☆
Security: ☆ ☆ ☆ ☆ ☆
Cleanliness: ☆ ☆ ☆ ☆ ☆

ADDRESS:	71 US 158 East Gatesville, NC 27938
OPERATED BY:	North Carolina State Parks
INFORMATION:	(252) 357-1191; ncparks.gov; reservations: (877) 722-6762
OPEN:	Year-round
SITES:	20
EACH SITE:	Picnic table, fire ring, lantern post, tent pad, trash can
ASSIGNMENT:	First come, first served and by reservation
REGISTRATION:	Ranger will come by to register you
FACILITIES:	Hot showers, flush toilets, water; showers on from mid-March to November
PARKING:	At campsites only
FEE:	$15
ELEVATION:	25 feet
RESTRICTIONS:	*Pets:* On leash only *Fires:* In fire rings only *Alcohol:* Prohibited *Vehicles:* No more than two per site *Other:* 14-day stay limit in 30-day period

Bennetts Creek was dammed more than 180 years ago, forming Merchants Millpond. The elevated pond provided waterpower to operate a gristmill and later a sawmill in Gates County. The 760-acre pond, ringed with cypress and gum trees, is filled with fish and other wildlife. Lassiter Swamp occupies the upper reaches of Bennetts Creek and the millpond. Canoes—for touring the swamp or casting a line to catch bream, crappie, or largemouth bass—are available for rent at very reasonable prices. Only electric motors are allowed on the lake, making it a quiet nature retreat. There are even backcountry canoe campsites for the adventurous. Check at the park office for canoe-rental information.

The park can also be explored by land. Several foot trails course through the woods and along the wetlands. One trail even has a campsite for backpackers. If you hike no other path, at least check out Cypress Point Trail, which makes a quarter-mile loop along the edge of the millpond, overlooking the swamp from a boardwalk. Coleman Trail extends 2 miles. It offers good views of the millpond, travels through several habitats, and is a good birding trail, especially during spring and fall migrations. Lassiter Trail, the master path of the park, can be picked up directly from the campground via a 0.4-mile spur trail. Make the 5-mile loop by passing along the north side of the millpond and along Lassiter Swamp. A park fire road cuts the loop in half. Park programs are held on weekends and will help inform you about this special swath of the coastal plain, which plainly, you should not miss.

MAP

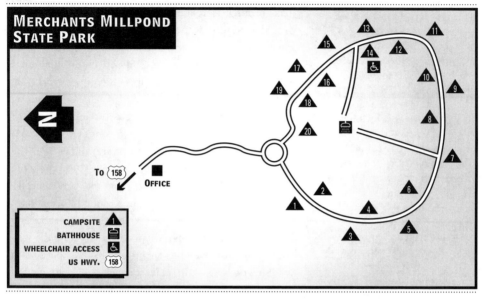

MERCHANTS MILLPOND STATE PARK

To 158
OFFICE

CAMPSITE
BATHHOUSE
WHEELCHAIR ACCESS
US HWY. 158

GETTING THERE

From Exit 173 on I-95, drive
east on US 158 61 miles to
the park, located on your
right, west of Sunbury.

GPS COORDINATES

UTM Zone (WGS84)	18S
Easting	0349570
Northing	4032730
Latitude	36 25' 47.7"
Longitude	76 40' 40.9"

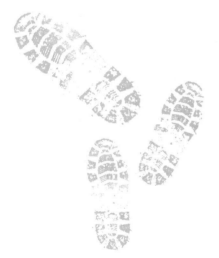

> *This national forest campground has received a face-lift.*

LOCALLY KNOWN AS FLANNERS BEACH, this revamped bluffside campground on the lower Neuse River is a fine recreation destination. The well-kept camp received a face-lift after storm damage from a series of hurricanes in the late 1990s, most notably Hurricane Fran in 1996. A paved hiking and biking trail loops through the campground. Flanners Beach, a sandy shoreline along the tidally influenced lower Neuse River, has been a swimming and water-side recreation destination for a long time.

The campground is laid out in a loop. As you pass the campground host, there for your security, tall loblolly pines reach for the sky above an understory of smaller oaks and sweetgums. You will immediately notice that the campground has a landscaped look, as opposed to random tree growth. Starting in 2000, brushy live oaks, willows, and many other trees were planted, especially between campsites to add privacy. Whether it returns to a completely natural look over time is irrelevant because the vegetation adds to the attractiveness of the Neuse River. More improvements are slated for the future, such as an additional loop just for tent campers. As it is, the first several campsites in the loop have electricity, attracting the big rigs. But let not your heart be troubled, as 33 out of 42 sites are nonelectric. The sites on the inside of the loop have more shade and vegetation than those on the outside, but they are smaller as well. A trip or two around the loop will reveal a mixture of sunny and shady spots. Several sites are close to the river, but the bluff prevents quick access to Flanners Beach. Sites are generally available on all but summer-holiday weekends, and always during the week. A modern bathhouse centers the loop and is easily accessible to all campers.

The area encompassing the Croatan National Forest has a long history. Its name was likely derived

RATINGS

Beauty: ✩ ✩ ✩ ✩
Privacy: ✩ ✩ ✩
Spaciousness: ✩ ✩ ✩ ✩
Quiet: ✩ ✩ ✩
Security: ✩ ✩ ✩ ✩
Cleanliness: ✩ ✩ ✩

from the Croatan people, who settled in villages along the Neuse River. The nearby town of New Bern, North Carolina's second oldest, was established in 1710. Timber from the area became important in the production of tar. Later, small farms were established but were bought out, along with larger holdings, to establish the Croatan National Forest in 1936 for timber management and watershed protection. Recreation areas were developed over the decades, including Neuse River Campground. An errant mapmaker decided to name the campground after the nearby Neuse River, but the name has never caught on, and locals call the area Flanners Beach to this day.

A paved recreation trail is open to bikes and hikers. It winds through the thick woods of the Neuse River bluff, about 30 feet above the river, and a tupelo swamp. A paved trail also connects the campground to an appealing picnic area where towering pines and hardwoods shade a grassy lawn. Wooden steps lead down to Flanners Beach. The tan sand, littered with driftwood, extends several yards in each direction, making for ample sunning and relaxing room (I enjoyed looking over the water here). No alcoholic beverages are allowed at the swim beach and picnic area.

The Neuse at this point is more of a bay than an inland river. Anglers can cast a line for striped bass, sunfish, largemouth bass, flounder, and crappie. The nearest boat ramp in the Croatan is at Cahooque Creek. Croatan National Forest offers other recreation opportunities on the tidal estuaries and freshwater lakes. Hikers can tackle the 26-mile Neusiok Trail, which crosses the 161,000-acre forest. On the way in to the campground, stop at the ranger station for more information. You can buy supplies back in New Bern.

KEY INFORMATION

ADDRESS: 141 East Fisher Ave. New Bern, NC 28560

OPERATED BY: U.S. Forest Service

INFORMATION: (252) 638-5628; cs.unca.edu/nfsnc

OPEN: Year-round

SITES: 44

EACH SITE: Picnic table, fire grate, lantern post; some sites have electricity

ASSIGNMENT: First come, first served; no reservations

REGISTRATION: Self-registration on site

FACILITIES: Hot showers, water spigots, flush toilets

PARKING: At campsites only

FEE: $15, $20 electric sites

ELEVATION: 30 feet

RESTRICTIONS: *Pets:* On leash only
Fires: In fire rings only
Alcohol: At campsites only
Vehicles: None
Other: 14-day stay limit

MAP

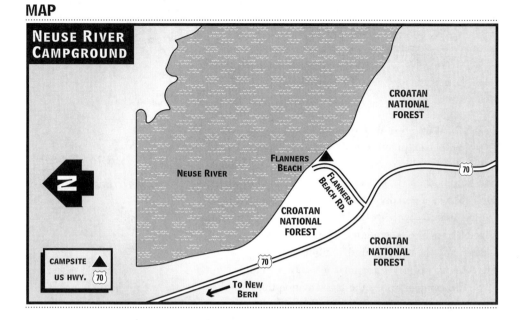

NEUSE RIVER CAMPGROUND

CROATAN NATIONAL FOREST

FLANNERS BEACH

NEUSE RIVER

FLANNERS BEACH RD.

70

CROATAN NATIONAL FOREST

CROATAN NATIONAL FOREST

CAMPSITE ▲
US HWY. 70

70

To NEW BERN

GETTING THERE

From New Bern, drive 12 miles east on US 70 to Flanners Beach Road, 2 miles beyond the Croatan Rangers Station, on your left. Turn left on Flanners Beach Road, and follow it 1.5 miles to reach the campground.

GPS COORDINATES

UTM Zone (WGS84) 18S
Easting 0322210
Northing 3872540
Latitude 34 58' 52.5"
Longitude 76 56' 51.0"

35
OCRACOKE ISLAND CAMPGROUND

OCRACOKE ISLAND is accessible only by ferry, but the extra effort reaps scenic rewards. Most of the island is part of the Cape Hatteras National Seashore and is kept in its natural state. The village of Ocracoke is a worthy destination. It evokes a 1950s fishing hamlet, with its cottages, narrow streets, and lack of franchise operations. The natural setting, the village, and the campground combine to make a relaxing getaway worth visiting for a few days or more.

The campground is the least inviting thing on the island, but it will suffice as your headquarters for exploring Ocracoke. The 137 campsites are in a flat behind dunes that separate you from the beach and the Atlantic Ocean. Most of the sites are on the main loop, which is broken by three crossroads; the sites on the inside of the loop are small and close together. Some small cedars and other trees, pruned back by the relentless wind, dot the otherwise-grassy campground. The loop curves around to reach the so-called dune sites, which are larger and are a short walk toward the beach from the paved parking pad. Other sites have average tent areas directly by the parking pad. Even the dune sites are open to the sun.

The loop curves away from the beach. The sites here, located away from the water but still an easy walk to the beach, back up to a wetland, which can be problematic if the mosquitoes are biting. The sites on the loop crossroads are mostly flat, grassy, and open to the sun. Three separate restroom areas with cold showers are spread throughout the campground.

Reservations can be made in advance, but you cannot pick out a specific site. A timely arrival is recommended even with a reservation, especially on weekends. Reservations can be made only between mid-May and mid-September, and are highly recommended on holiday weekends and from early July

> *This island campground is accessible only by car ferry.*

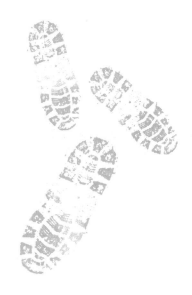

RATINGS

Beauty: ☆ ☆ ☆
Privacy: ☆
Spaciousness: ☆ ☆
Quiet: ☆ ☆ ☆ ☆ ☆
Security: ☆ ☆ ☆ ☆
Cleanliness: ☆ ☆ ☆

ADDRESS: 4352 Irvin Garrish Hwy. Ocracoke, NC 27960

OPERATED BY: National Park Service

INFORMATION: (252) 473-2111; nps.gov/caha; reservations: (877) 444-6777, recreation.gov; ferry information: (800) 293-3779, ncferry.org

OPEN: Friday of Easter weekend– mid-October

SITES: 136

EACH SITE: Picnic table, upright grill

ASSIGNMENT: First come, first served and by reservation mid-May– mid-September

REGISTRATION: At campground entrance booth

FACILITIES: Cold showers, water spigots, flush toilets

PARKING: At campsites only

FEE: $23

ELEVATION: 20 feet

RESTRICTIONS: *Pets:* On leash only *Fires:* In upright grills only *Alcohol:* At campsites only *Vehicles:* Must be parked on paved surface

through mid-August. Be aware that mosquitoes can be a problem after wet spells, so mosquito repellent and a screen shelter will make your stay much more enjoyable. Furthermore, if you are taking the Cedar Island ferry or the Swan Quarter ferry, it's also wise to make reservations for your arrival and departure, especially during the busy season. I recommend coming during the shoulder seasons, when the crowds are gone, the village of Ocracoke is in really low gear, and the better campsites are available.

Life is slow on Ocracoke Island. You can sense it as you walk the beach. A great place for quiet walks is the beach-access area across from the pony pens (more about those later). No cars are allowed on the beach here, and no development can be seen. (Cars are allowed on the beach near the campground.) Sea kayaking is popular on the Pamlico Sound side of the island, and boats of all sorts can be rented in the village of Ocracoke (supplies can be purchased here as well). You can also rent bikes for pedaling around the village, charter a sport-fishing boat, eat in a unique restaurant (no franchises allowed!), visit the Ocracoke Lighthouse (built in the early 1800s), or just sit back on a bench at Silver Lake Harbor and watch the boats come and go. Take the Ocracoke Historical Interpretive Trail to learn about the lengthy past of this land. This place really does have character.

The ponies that once roamed Ocracoke are now taken care of by the park service. They are quartered a few miles from the campground. The animals are thought to have swum ashore from a Spanish shipwreck long ago. An interpretive trail travels near the horse pens. Another interpretive trail, Hardwood Hammocks Trail, travels into the island interior. The path starts just across the road from the campground. Start your planning now for a trip to Ocracoke Island.

MAP

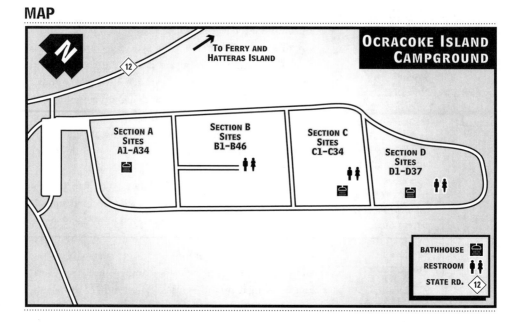

OCRACOKE ISLAND CAMPGROUND

TO FERRY AND HATTERAS ISLAND

12

SECTION A
SITES
A1–A34

SECTION B
SITES
B1–B46

SECTION C
SITES
C1–C34

SECTION D
SITES
D1–D37

BATHHOUSE
RESTROOM
STATE RD. 12

GPS COORDINATES

UTM Zone (WGS84) 18S

Easting 0410450

Northing 3880650

Latitude 35 7' 36.9"

Longitude 75 55' 8.7"

GETTING THERE

From the intersection of US 64/264 and US 158 just south of Nags Head, drive south on NC 12 59 miles to the ferry at the southwest end of Hatteras Island. From here, take the free ferry over to Ocracoke Island. Once off the ferry, keep south on NC 12 9.5 miles to reach the campground, on your left. Two other, longer toll-ferry options reach Ocracoke Island as well; for more information, call (800) 293-3779.

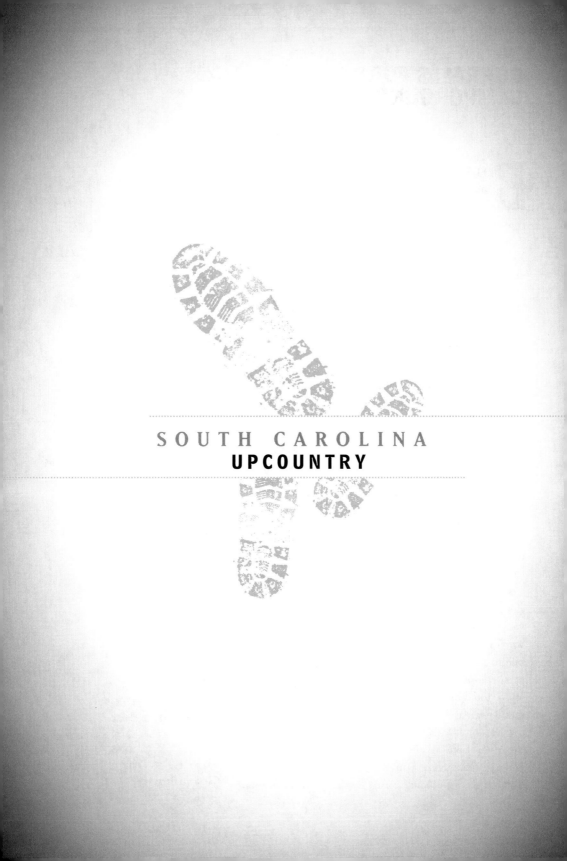

SOUTH CAROLINA
UPCOUNTRY

36
BURRELLS FORD
CAMPGROUND

BEFORE THE CHATTOOGA was declared a Wild and Scenic River, campers could drive all the way to Burrells Ford Campground. Since then, a protective corridor has been established, effectively cutting off direct auto access to the campground. This has had mixed results: it has limited the use of the campground but has cut maintenance as well. The short walk may deter some tent campers, but you can guarantee that no RVs will ever be at Burrells Ford.

Follow the old jeep road down to the river, entering the protected corridor. The road forks at the river bottom, forested in tall white pines, with a thick understory of holly trees, rhododendrons, and mountain laurels. The Chattooga runs shallow and clear directly in front of the campground—no doubt the ford of days gone by. On the other side of the river, deeply shaded in thick, junglelike vegetation, lies the state of Georgia. Deep pools lie both upstream and downstream of the campground, beckoning the camper to drop a line or take a dip. Rainbow and brown trout thrive in the mountain water.

The right fork of the old jeep road leads directly to the Chattooga. Campsites are spread along both sides of the road. Most are cooled beneath the shady canopy, but some lie in a glade that receives enough sun for grass to grow. All the sites offer maximum privacy, as they are well away from one another. You won't be able to carry enough stuff from your automobile to the campground to use all the space offered at each campsite, although on my visit, one enterprising fellow toted his belongings down from the parking area in a wheelbarrow.

The left fork of the road enters the south side of the river bottom after crossing the clear and cool Kings Creek. Here you'll find more primitive sites: usually just a flat spot, a fire ring, and an occasional

> *The Chattooga River and Ellicott Rock Wilderness are just a few footsteps away from this primitive campground.*

RATINGS

Beauty: ✩ ✩ ✩ ✩
Privacy: ✩ ✩ ✩ ✩ ✩
Spaciousness: ✩ ✩ ✩ ✩ ✩
Quiet: ✩ ✩ ✩ ✩ ✩
Security: ✩ ✩ ✩
Cleanliness: ✩ ✩ ✩

KEY INFORMATION

ADDRESS: 112 Andrew Pickens Cir. Mountain Rest, SC 29664

OPERATED BY: U.S. Forest Service

INFORMATION: (864) 638-9568; fs.fed.us/r8/fms

OPEN: Year-round

SITES: Not designated, but there is room for 9 tents

EACH SITE: Picnic table, fire ring, lantern post

ASSIGNMENT: First come, first served; no reservations

REGISTRATION: Not necessary

FACILITIES: Hand-pumped water, pit toilet

PARKING: At Burrells Ford parking area

FEE: None

ELEVATION: 2,000 feet

RESTRICTIONS: *Pets:* On leash only
Fires: In fire rings only
Alcohol: At campsites only
Vehicles: In parking area only; no RVs or trailers
Other: No trash cans—pack it in, pack it out; campers must carry tents one-third of a mile to site

picnic table or lantern post. In a nearby flat, just upstream on Kings Creek, a very isolated site backs up against a steep hill for the tent camper seeking the ultimate in privacy. The left fork of the road intersects the Foothills Trail along the river; here, you'll encounter many secluded and flat campsites. Solitude is yours, to say the least.

Burrells Ford is rustic, and, as expected, amenities are minimal. After all, it is within a Wild and Scenic River corridor and borders the Ellicott Rock Wilderness. Your arms will get a workout at the hand-pump well near the head of the campground. Two pit toilets are available for your basic comfort.

To see more of the attractive riverine ecosystem of the Chattooga, you only need to choose whether to go up or down the river. Down the Chattooga is the Foothills Trail. It winds along the river past Big Bend Falls for some 5 miles to Licklog Creek before turning southeast toward Oconee State Park. You can keep south along the river 4.8 miles on the Chattooga Trail to Ridley Fields and SC 28. But first, tune up with a short 0.3-mile hike up Kings Creek to a woodsy waterfall, then return to camp.

Upstream and north from Burrells Ford, Foothills Trail climbs away from the river along Medlin Mountain on its journey to Table Rock State Park nearly 70 miles away. If you stay north along the river, you'll soon enter the 7,000-acre Ellicott Rock Wilderness on the north section of the Chattooga Trail, which leads 4 scenic miles past riverside beaches to Ellicott Rock. This spot was selected in 1811 by a surveyor named Andrew Ellicott to designate the exact location where the Carolinas and Georgia came together. Ellicott chiseled "NC" in 1811 on this trailside marker. The actual point at which the three states meet is Commissioner's Rock, extending into the Chattooga River a few feet distant. Stand here and you can be in three states at once. Take the short side of the trail to Spoon Auger Falls on your way back.

It takes a little effort to reach Burrells Ford Campground, but you will be well rewarded. The Chattooga deserves its Wild and Scenic status, and the surrounding mountain lands are wild and scenic as well.

MAP

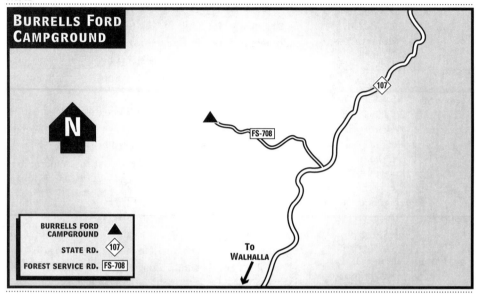

BURRELLS FORD CAMPGROUND

N

BURRELLS FORD CAMPGROUND	▲
STATE RD.	107
FOREST SERVICE RD.	FS-708

FS-708

107

To
WALHALLA

GETTING THERE

From Walhalla, drive north
on SC 28 8.5 miles to
SC 107; then turn right.
Follow SC 107 8.9 miles.
Then turn left on gravel
Forest Service Road 708.
Descend on FS 708 3 miles.
Burrells Ford parking area
will be on your left.

GPS COORDINATES

UTM Zone (WGS84) 17S
Easting 0306857
Northing 3871736
Latitude 34 58' 17.8"
Longitude 83 6' 56.4"

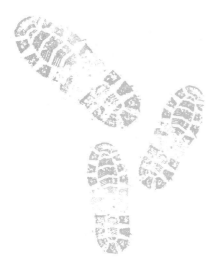

Cherry Hill is South Carolina's finest upcountry campground.

CHERRY HILL CAMPGROUND is the focal point for the Cherry Hill Recreation Area. And as one of the best national forest campgrounds in the Southern Appalachians, it is a fine place to be. The campground, in the shallow upper valley of West Fork Creek, lies covered with an abundant understory beneath a towering forest of hardwood and pine. The U.S. Forest Service must work hard to keep the vegetation from reclaiming this land.

Just off SC 107 is the entrance to the campground. Immediately to the left is a circular turnaround, known as the overflow area. It once was home to a settler, whose chimney still stands just off the loop; a short path leads to the ruins. Four campsites have been carved into the woods there, but you must park on the loop and carry your belongings a few feet to the new sites.

The main campground lies beyond the overflow area on a short spur road that descends to tranquil West Fork Creek. Just past the self-service pay station are two sites isolated on their own mini-loop. A water spigot is nearby. Three other sites are off the spur road before you reach the main loop, which makes a large oval beside the West Fork.

All the sites along the West Fork are shrouded in rhododendron and are ideal for campers who like deep, lush woods. Four relatively open sites are on the inside of the main loop and offer a generous amount of space for even the most gear-laden camper. The sites away from the West Fork back against a hill beneath more open woods. Three water spigots are situated throughout the main loop. A clean, well-kept comfort station is at the north end of the loop; it has warm showers and flush toilets. There are no electric hookups.

Near the comfort station, a small circular drive splits off the main loop. It holds four campsites with large parking areas, apparently designed for RVers,

RATINGS

Beauty: ✿ ✿ ✿ ✿ ✿
Privacy: ✿ ✿ ✿ ✿
Spaciousness: ✿ ✿ ✿ ✿ ✿
Quiet: ✿ ✿ ✿ ✿ ✿
Security: ✿ ✿ ✿ ✿
Cleanliness: ✿ ✿ ✿ ✿ ✿

who were the only campers I saw at that spot during my visit. The circle has its own water spigot.

A campground host is stationed at Cherry Hill and keeps the place immaculate and safe. This only adds to the relaxing atmosphere of the area. Just as you get really comfortable, a notion will strike you to venture beyond your folding chair to explore more of the beauty of Sumter National Forest. And you don't even have to leave Cherry Hill to walk some of the area trails. For starters, try Cherry Hill Nature Trail. It leaves the campground and makes a half-mile loop among the ferns and brush of the white-pine forest.

Winding Stairs Trail also leaves from the campground. Follow it down as it switchbacks through an oak forest along the south side of the West Fork. I can only guess that the gentle switchbacking led to the Winding Stairs name. At any rate, after a mile, you'll come to a small but steep waterfall, as West Fork Creek has picked up some volume on its way to merge with Crane Creek. After the fall, Winding Stairs Trail veers south to Crane Creek, then returns to West Fork only to end at 3.5 miles on Forest Service Road 710.

If you want bigger water, the Chattooga, a Wild and Scenic River, is only a stroll away on Big Bend Trail. The trail starts just across SC 107 from the campground and leads 2.7 miles west into the protected corridor of the Chattooga 0.8 miles upstream of Big Bend Falls. From there, trails lead along the river in both directions for miles. Either way you go, you'll soon understand why this border river between South Carolina and Georgia is protected. The flora, fauna, and tumbling white water are yours to appreciate. The fishing's good, too.

Cherry Hill is a great campground in an attractive forest setting. And for $10, it is a superlative value. Get all your supplies back in Walhalla, because once you're at Cherry Hill, you won't want to spoil your vacation with an early return to civilization.

KEY INFORMATION

ADDRESS:	112 Andrew Pickens Cir. Mountain Rest, SC 29664
OPERATED BY:	U.S. Forest Service
INFORMATION:	(864) 638-9568; fs.fed.us/r8/fms
OPEN:	April–October
SITES:	29
EACH SITE:	Picnic table, fire pit, lantern post
ASSIGNMENT:	First come, first served; no reservations
REGISTRATION:	Self-registration on site
FACILITIES:	Water, flush toilets, hot showers
PARKING:	At campsites only
FEE:	$10
ELEVATION:	2,250 feet
RESTRICTIONS:	*Pets:* On leash only *Fires:* In fire pits only *Alcohol:* At campsites only *Vehicles:* None *Other:* No more than six campers per site; tents in designated areas only

MAP

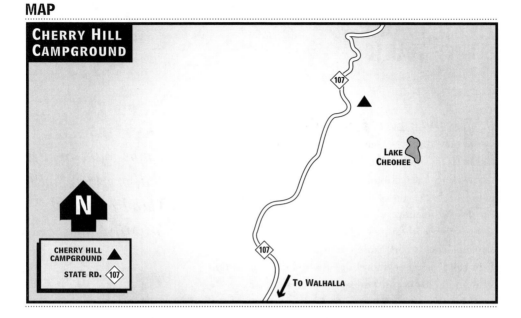

CHERRY HILL CAMPGROUND

107

LAKE CHEOHEE

N

CHERRY HILL CAMPGROUND ▲

STATE RD. 107

107

To Walhalla

GETTING THERE

From Walhalla, drive north on SC 28 8.5 miles to SC 107; then turn right. Follow SC 107 7.5 miles. The entrance to Cherry Hill Campground will be on your right.

GPS COORDINATES

UTM Zone (WGS84) 17S
Easting 0309190
Northing 3868400
Latitude 34 56' 33.6"
Longitude 83 5' 16.8"

38
DEVILS FORK
STATE PARK

HAVE YOU EVER SEEN Lake Jocassee? Others may disagree, but I believe this impoundment to be South Carolina's most beautiful lake. A richly forested shoreline overlooks emerald water against a backdrop of the Blue Ridge Mountains. On the lake's northern shores are the Jocassee Gorges, steep valleys where waterfalls are fed by cool, clear streams. Devils Fork State Park occupies some of Lake Jocassee's awesome shoreline, abutted by walk-in tent sites and affording instant water access.

> *Enjoy walk-in sites that overlook South Carolina's most beautiful lake.*

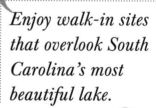

Being a water-oriented park, the campground is, unsurprisingly, near the shoreline. Even better, the walk-in tent sites are close to the lake. The main tent-camping area spurs onto a wooded peninsula extending into the lake, with a paved trail leading down to the campsites. Descend along a rib ridge covered in mountain laurels, oaks, pines, and tulip trees. Sites T-1 through T-8 dip toward the lake but are closer to the parking area. The mountain slope has been leveled at each site. Sites T-9 through T-15 overlook the water and offer a view of the mountains beyond the lake. Landscaping timbers have been installed at the sites and beyond to slow erosion. Sites T-16 through T-19 are too close to one another but overlook the lake; T-18 is the best of this bunch. Site T-20 is closest to the walk-in parking area. The least appealing sites here are T-6, T-8, and T-19, but they are still better than most sites at other campgrounds. A water spigot lies at the beginning of the walk-in-camper access trail.

A second set of walk-in tent sites is accessible from the day-use area, near a playground. Take a short gravel path to reach sites T-21 through T-25, where the woods are more open. Site T-22 is near the lake. Sites T-23 and T-24 are a little too close together. Site T-25 has the farthest walk but ends up near some of the

RATINGS

Beauty: ☆ ☆ ☆ ☆
Privacy: ☆ ☆ ☆
Spaciousness: ☆ ☆ ☆
Quiet: ☆ ☆ ☆
Security: ☆ ☆ ☆ ☆ ☆
Cleanliness: ☆ ☆ ☆ ☆

ADDRESS: 161 Holcombe Cir.
Salem, SC 29676

OPERATED BY: South Carolina
State Parks

INFORMATION: (864) 944-2639;
southcarolina
parks.com;
reservations:
(866) 345-7275,
reserve
america.com

OPEN: Year-round

SITES: 25 walk-in tent
sites, 59 others

EACH SITE: Walk-in tent sites
have picnic table,
fire ring, tent pad;
other sites also
have water and
electricity

ASSIGNMENT: First come,
first served and
by reservation

REGISTRATION: At park office

FACILITIES: Hot showers, flush
toilets, water spig-
ots, laundry

PARKING: At walk-in parking area and at
campsites

FEE: $14–$15 walk-in
sites, $18–$20
others

ELEVATION: 1,150 feet

RESTRICTIONS: *Pets:* On leash only
Fires: In fire rings
only
Alcohol: Prohibited
Vehicles: No more
than two per site
Other: No more
than six campers
per walk-in site

drive-up sites in the main campground area. A water spigot is near these sites.

The main drive-up campground has two loops. Trees shade the sites, and ample vegetation screens them from one another. Most have tent pads. Any of these sites will suffice, but the tent sites are far more desirable. And because all sites are reservable, why not go for the ones you like? Reservations are strongly recommended, as the campground fills nearly every weekend from Easter through fall.

This park is fairly small but has two hiking trails. The 1.5-mile Oconee Bells Nature Trail takes you by places where the rare Oconee bell wildflower grows. Bear Cove Trail makes a 3.5-mile loop and starts at the day-use area. Most recreation centers on this beautiful lake. You'll see campers swimming near their sites, as no supervised swim area exists. Watercraft access to the lake is made easy at the park boat ramp. If you don't have a boat or you want to get shuttled across the lake to explore some of the Jocassee Gorges, Hoyett's Bait and Tackle is just outside the park. They have fishing gear and bait, rent boats, and offer shuttles and guided sightseeing and fishing tours on Lake Jocassee. Call them at (864) 944-9016.

Lake Jocassee is worth seeing. You can check out all the rivers that feed it from gorges coming out of the mountains—Whitewater River, Devils Fork Creek, Horsepasture River, and Toxaway River. I have explored them via Foothills Trail, which runs along the north shore of Lake Jocassee, and proclaim them a prize resource of both North and South Carolina. Make a reservation to tent camp at Devils Fork and explore Lake Jocassee; then see if you too think it is South Carolina's most beautiful lake.

MAP

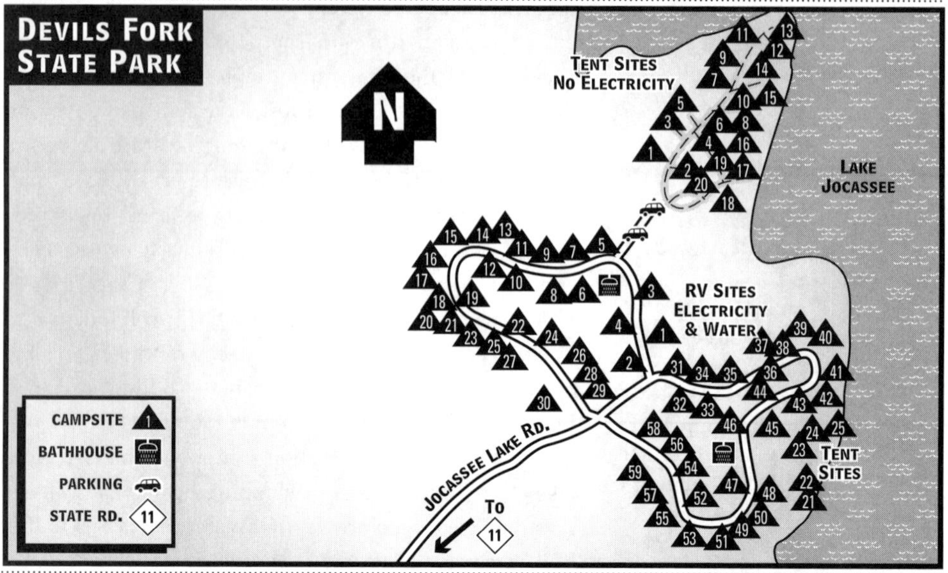

DEVILS FORK STATE PARK

N

TENT SITES NO ELECTRICITY

LAKE JOCASSEE

RV SITES ELECTRICITY & WATER

TENT SITES

JOCASSEE LAKE RD.

To 11

CAMPSITE
BATHHOUSE
PARKING
STATE RD. 11

GETTING THERE

From Pickens, drive on US 178 north 9 miles to SC 11. Turn left on SC 11, and follow it 12.5 miles to reach Jocassee Lake Road. Turn right on Jocassee Lake Road, and follow it 3.5 miles to reach the park.

GPS COORDINATES

UTM Zone (WGS84) 17S

Easting 0320940

Northing 3865940

Latitude 34 57' 28.9"

Longitude 82 57' 14.0"

> *South Carolina operates this ecological treasure more sensitively than most other state parks.*

THIS STATE PARK and the adjacent Caesars Head State Park are operated as low-impact wilderness parks. This means that they are not designed like traditional parks with big drive-up campgrounds, parking lots, and heavy usage areas. Rather, the park facilities are integrated into an exceptional mountain landscape, leaving the emphasis on the natural. Foot trails lead along crystalline streams crashing over mossy boulders beneath cathedral-like forests, where rock faces offer sweeping vistas and spring wildflowers peek through leaves that colored the landscape the previous fall.

For tent campers, "low impact" means carrying your stuff to rustic walk-in tent campsites and treading lightly on the land. It means packing your trash not only from your campsite but also from the entire park. It also means giving in to the spell the park puts on you, so that no matter what time of year you visit, it will make you want to return for more hiking through the Mountain Bridge Wilderness and for taking in more of the sights.

Jones Gap State Park offers 29 campsites. The nine described below are walk-in sites within a half mile of the camper parking area. The other 20 are considered backcountry campsites. To reach the walk-in sites, leave the camper parking area and cross a bridge over the Middle Saluda River, deservedly South Carolina's first designated scenic river. Ahead is the impressive log cabin that houses the park office and environmental learning center; this is where you register. If no one is there, use the nearby pay phone and call the pager number listed on the park office door. A ranger will come and assist you.

Now to the campsites, which are marked with green plastic posts. Sites 1 through 4 are located past the old fish-hatchery pool on Hospital Rock Trail, to

RATINGS

Beauty: ☆ ☆ ☆ ☆ ☆
Privacy: ☆ ☆ ☆ ☆
Spaciousness: ☆ ☆ ☆
Quiet: ☆ ☆ ☆ ☆ ☆
Security: ☆ ☆ ☆ ☆ ☆
Cleanliness: ☆ ☆ ☆ ☆

your right as you face the log cabin. The paved trail leads to a dirt trail and the woods. Site 1 is along a small streamlet among boulders in dark rhododendron. Site 2 is a little on the sloped side and is shaded by oaks. Site 3 is away from the water in a notch between two ridgelines, shaded by hickories and oaks. Site 4 is near the pipeline that feeds the hatchery pool and overlooks a mountain ravine.

Sites 5 through 7 are closest to the camper parking area. These lead into woods from a path just to the left of the log cabin, with the Middle Saluda nearby. Site 5 is up a hill on a neat, rocky flat. The numerous embedded boulders there act as camp furniture. Site 6 is in a flat directly beside the river. Site 7 is at the end of this short trail, fewer than 100 yards from the log-cabin office. It is banked against a hillside near the river, shaded by rhododendron.

Sites 8 and 9 are up the Jones Gap Trail heading directly up the Middle Saluda from the camper parking area. Site 8 is large and surrounded by hardwoods. The noise of the river crashing over boulders will sing you to sleep. Site 9 is the hardest to reach, 0.4 miles from the parking area. It is large, too, and is also along the river. Rocks and sand form the site's floor.

The campsites fill on the first nice weekends in spring, and then taper off when the heat rises. From mid-August until the leaves fall, the campsites can fill any weekend. During the week you can get a campsite anytime. The bathhouse, with a water spigot outside, is located near the log cabin. Be aware that the showers are open only from 6 p.m. to 8 a.m.

The picnic area near the log cabin and former hatchery area exudes tranquility. The mown grass contrasts with the verdant forests, steep mountains, and crashing river. You will wish you had a scenically located log cabin of your own. But visiting Jones Gap State Park is about hiking and exploring the Mountain Bridge Wilderness. Trails galore wind through the campground. One of my fondest outdoor memories occurred at Jones Gap. I hiked the entire Foothills Trail from Oconee State Park 90 miles to the park in fall. The final morning dawned cool and crisp as wood smoke curled from my fire. I walked down through

KEY INFORMATION

ADDRESS:	303 Jones Gap Rd. Marietta, SC 29661
OPERATED BY:	South Carolina State Parks
INFORMATION:	(864) 836-3647; southcarolina parks.com
OPEN:	Year-round
SITES:	9 walk-in sites
EACH SITE:	Fire grate
ASSIGNMENT:	First come, first served; no reservations
REGISTRATION:	At log cabin ranger station
FACILITIES:	Hot showers, flush toilets, water spigot
PARKING:	At walk-in-camper parking area
FEE:	$8–$20 depending on season
ELEVATION:	1,500 feet
RESTRICTIONS:	*Pets:* On leash only *Fires:* In fire rings only *Alcohol:* Prohibited *Vehicles:* No more than two per site *Other:* No trash cans—pack it in, pack it out

MAP

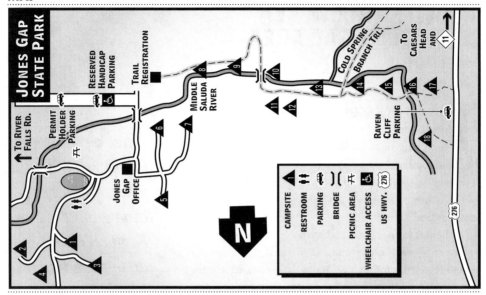

GETTING THERE

From Pickens, take SC 8 north 15 miles to SC 11. Veer right onto SC 11, and follow it 2 miles to US 276. Turn right on US 276, and follow it 4 miles to River Falls Road. Turn left on River Falls Road, and keep forward 5.5 miles as it turns into Jones Gap Road to dead-end at Jones Gap State Park.

GPS COORDINATES

UTM Zone (WGS84) 17S
Easting 0356690
Northing 3887860
Latitude 35 7' 35.3"
Longitude 82 34' 20.6"

The Winds (as in winding a clock) along the numerous cascades of the Middle Saluda. Framed in autumn color, I enjoyed the satisfaction of completing the entire trail with such an inspiring ending.

Jones Gap has many other trails and destinations in addition to the river. The combined area of Jones Gap and adjacent Caesars Head state parks is known as the Mountain Bridge Wilderness Area. A wilderness trail map, available at the park office, reveals much more than a weekend's worth of possibilities. Head to Raven Cliff Falls or Hospital Rock, or hike up Cold Spring Branch to enjoy wildflowers. A shorter but challenging loop includes the Rim of the Gap Trail and returns via Little Pinnacle Mountain on the Pinnacle Pass Trail. Jones Gap is all about trails and wilderness; just remember to leave the land in this mountain treasure the way you found it.

40
KEOWEE-TOXAWAY STATE NATURAL AREA

THIS AREA OF SOUTH CAROLINA is aptly named the Cherokee Foothills. The Cherokee thrived here long before white settlers ever laid eyes on the land. South Carolina recognizes this, and Keowee-Toxaway celebrates native culture in the natural setting of the Cherokee Foothills at this quiet, well-maintained state natural area.

Tent campers can enjoy the area by day and return to a great campground at night. It is situated on a well-wooded knoll that tastefully integrates campsites with the steep terrain using well-placed landscaping timbers. Shade is abundant beneath the canopy of hickories and oaks, though a relatively light understory somewhat diminishes privacy.

Tent campers have their own separate loop. No loud generators will interfere with the sounds of chirping birds. The 14 tent sites are all spacious and level enough for setting up a normal amount of gear, but expect some seriously sloping topography if you stray from your designated area. That slope, though, allows for balcony-like views into the hollows beyond the campground knoll. The sites on the inside of the loop are less steep beyond their timbered camping area. The tent pads at this state park are among the finest I have seen—they are slightly crowned in the center, allowing for quick runoff during those heavy mountain thunderstorms. This is just one more obvious sign that the campground is well designed.

Another plus is that you'll never have to go far for water. Three spigots are evenly distributed along the small loop. RVers and tent campers share a comfort station located between the two separate loops. Hot showers and flush toilets are provided. Additional features include firewood for sale at the park office and excellent campground safety. In fact, this might be the safest campground in the state. Park gates are locked at

Cherokee heritage, scenic hill country, mountain lakes, and a peaceful campground make Keowee-Toxaway an outstanding state natural area.

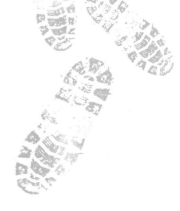

RATINGS

Beauty: ✩ ✩ ✩ ✩
Privacy: ✩ ✩ ✩ ✩
Spaciousness: ✩ ✩ ✩ ✩
Quiet: ✩ ✩ ✩ ✩
Security: ✩ ✩ ✩ ✩ ✩
Cleanliness: ✩ ✩ ✩ ✩ ✩

ADDRESS:	108 Residence Dr. Sunset, SC 29685
OPERATED BY:	South Carolina State Parks
INFORMATION:	(864) 868-2605; southcarolina parks.com; reservations: (866) 345-7275, reserve america.com
OPEN:	Year-round
SITES:	14 tent-only sites, 10 RV sites
EACH SITE:	Tent pad, picnic table, fire ring with attached grill
ASSIGNMENT:	First come, first served and by reservation
REGISTRATION:	Ranger will come by to register you
FACILITIES:	Water, flush toilets, hot showers
PARKING:	At campsites only
FEE:	$8–$10, $12–$14 RV sites, depending on season
ELEVATION:	1,000 feet
RESTRICTIONS:	*Pets:* On leash only *Fires:* In fire rings only *Alcohol:* Prohibited *Vehicles:* None *Other:* 14-day stay limit on one campsite

night, and the ranger residence is just a stone's throw away from the tenters' loop.

Near the park office is Keowee-Toxaway's centerpiece: the Cherokee Interpretive Center, which recognizes the area's Cherokee heritage. During my visit I learned quite a bit about native life before, during, and after the arrival of European settlers, and also about the flora and fauna that inhabit the state park. Visit the interpretive center first for an enhanced appreciation of the historic and natural life here.

Just outside the interpretive center is the quarter-mile Cherokee Interpretive Trail. It winds through the woods and chronicles the evolution of the Cherokee tribe at four informative kiosks, culminating with the story of their removal from their ancestral lands along the infamous Trail of Tears.

Other, longer trails carpet the park. The 4-mile Raven Rock Trail undulates amid the piney hills and hardwood hollows along clear creeks to a rock cliff overlooking Lake Keowee, then loops back via the Natural Bridge Trail to the park's Meeting House. A rock bridge spans Poe Creek along the Natural Bridge Trail. The 0.7-mile Lake Trail leads from the campground down to the shore of Lake Keowee. This natural area may be only 1,000 acres, but South Carolinians make the most of the scenic beauty packed into the small package.

Lake lovers have two nearby bodies of water to enjoy. Both Lake Keowee and Lake Jocassee back against the Blue Ridge, affording mountainous shorelines. Lake Keowee, the larger of the two, is a warm-water fishery, with bass and bream as its primary sport fish. Anglers will be surprised to find trout in Lake Jocassee's deep, cool waters. Nearby Devils Fork State Park is on Lake Jocassee and offers good camping as well, with a special section of walk-in tent sites.

Overall, you will find the understated Keowee-Toxaway State Natural Area a pleasant surprise. It is ideal for tent campers who want an intimate, well-kept campground with plenty of amenities. The blending of Cherokee heritage and natural beauty was a masterstroke by South Carolina park officials. Don't make the mistake of overlooking this small jewel of the Palmetto State.

MAP

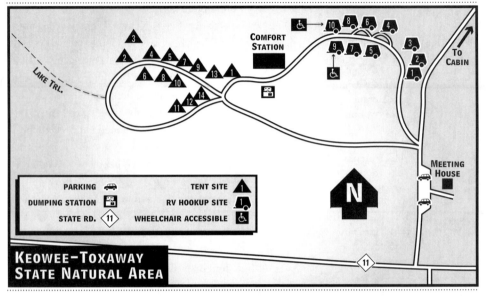

COMFORT
STATION

TO
CABIN

LAKE TRL.

MEETING
HOUSE

N

PARKING

DUMPING STATION

STATE RD. 11

TENT SITE

RV HOOKUP SITE

WHEELCHAIR ACCESSIBLE

KEOWEE-TOXAWAY
STATE NATURAL AREA

11

GETTING THERE

From Pickens drive north on
US 178 9 miles to SC 11.
Turn left on SC 11, and
drive 7.9 miles to Keowee-
Toxaway State Park.

GPS COORDINATES

UTM Zone (WGS84) 17S

Easting 0327500

Northing 3867090

Latitude 34 56' 1.0"

Longitude 82 53' 18.9"

> *Oconee State Park is one example of the fine recreation destinations in South Carolina's Golden Corner.*

LOCATED IN OCONEE COUNTY, also known as South Carolina's Golden Corner, Oconee State Park is perched at 1,800 feet in the Blue Ridge Mountains, offering a cool place to camp during the long, hot summer. But the park offers much more than that. For starters, the walk-in tent-camping sites stack up to any others in the state and make the park's other campsites pale in comparison. The mountain terrain features great hiking, especially when you add in the trails of Sumter National Forest, which borders much of the park. The much-touted Foothills Trail begins here, marching 76 miles to Table Rock State Park or alternatively to Jones Gap State Park. Oconee State Park has two lakes for fishing and swimming. Nearby, the federally designated Wild and Scenic Chattooga River has outfitters ready to take you on guided white-water trips.

The walk-in tent sites spur from the main campground near site 70. A pair of carts aids in toting gear back to the sites from the parking area. Leave the walk-in parking area on a footpath. A scenic mountain forest of maple, hickory, oak, and white pine grows overhead. Smaller trees, mountain laurel, and cane grow as an understory. The trail splits, and sites T-1 through T-10 are ahead. The hillside sites have been leveled, and all are well shaded and private, especially T-7. Site T-8 was my pick. Beyond site T-10, the walk-in access trail keeps forward to meet the Oconee Trail.

Sites T-11 through T-15 are farther from the parking area. Follow a common path before reaching a level area, where spur trails lead downhill to the sites, which are near the park's smaller lake. Site T-11 is in a thicket of mountain laurel. Site T-12, also in mountain laurel, is closer to the lake. A small path leads to the water. T-13 has room to roam. T-14 is close to the water and is well

RATINGS

Beauty: ✫ ✫ ✫ ✫
Privacy: ✫ ✫ ✫
Spaciousness: ✫ ✫ ✫ ✫
Quiet: ✫ ✫ ✫ ✫
Security: ✫ ✫ ✫ ✫ ✫
Cleanliness: ✫ ✫ ✫ ✫

shaded by white pines. T-15, the most private of them all, is the farthest from the parking area.

The main campground may scare you. The sites are mostly small and crowded, but they do have water and electricity. A hard look around may yield a few nice sites, but overall these don't begin to compare with the walk-in tent sites. I would rather not stay here if I couldn't get a walk-in tent site, which is most likely a problem on holiday weekends. The main campground does have a recreation building handy for rainy days. The Trading Post, a small camp store, is open during the warm season. Sites should be available most weekends, other than holidays, and all weekdays. The last two weekends in October see an upsurge in traffic from leaf watchers.

Oddly, a miniature-golf course abuts the campground and is the only artificial diversion around. The lakes are a nicer recreational alternative than mini-golf, but the mountains and trails running over them are the real attraction. At the lakes, the park rents johnboats, canoes, kayaks, and paddleboats for tooling around or fishing for catfish, bream, and bass (no private boats are allowed). Trout are stocked here during winter, and a swim area is on the larger lake.

It only seems fitting that this lake would have a trail around it—Lake Trail—since this park is very trail oriented. Old Waterwheel Trail leads to the site where the Civilian Conservation Corps, which originally developed the park in the 1930s, built a waterwheel to pump water. Hidden Falls Trail leads to a 60-foot waterfall. Start your hike to the falls on the Foothills Trail, which leads down to the Chattooga River and beyond. Tamassee Knob Trail also spurs from Foothills Trail. Here, you reach a rock outcrop with far-reaching views to the west. You can actually connect to all these trails, except Lake Trail, from Oconee Trail, which runs directly by the walk-in camping area. A trail map is available at the park office, where you can see some neat relics from the CCC days.

If you haven't rafted the Chattooga, here's your chance. The river is fewer than 10 miles away, and several outfitters are in the vicinity. The park office has a list of outfitters and directions to the Chattooga. This

KEY INFORMATION

ADDRESS: 624 State Park Rd. Mountain Rest, SC 29664

OPERATED BY: South Carolina State Parks

INFORMATION: (864) 638-5353; southcarolina parks.com; reservations: (866) 345-7275, reserve america.com

OPEN: Year-round

SITES: 15 walk-in tent sites, 140 others

EACH SITE: Walk-in sites have picnic tables, fire grates, tent pads, lantern posts; other sites also have water and electricity

ASSIGNMENT: First come, first served and by reservation; walk-in tent sites are first come, first served only

REGISTRATION: At campground trading post if open; otherwise, ranger will come by to register you

FACILITIES: Hot showers, flush toilets, water spigots, camp store in season

PARKING: At walk-in-camper parking area and at campsites

FEE: $12–$13 walk-in sites, $16–$18 other sites

ELEVATION: 1,825 feet

RESTRICTIONS: *Pets:* On leash only *Fires:* In fire rings only *Alcohol:* Prohibited *Vehicles:* No more than two per site *Other:* 14-day stay limit

MAP

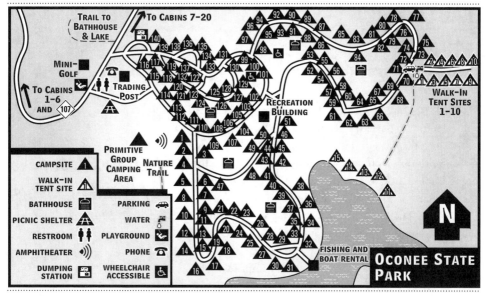

GETTING THERE

From Walhalla, drive north on SC 28 north 8.5 miles to SC 107. Turn right on SC 107, and follow it 2.5 miles to the state park, on your right.

has been one of my favorite rivers for a long time, be it for backpacking, fishing, tent camping, or rafting. You might say the Chattooga River and Oconee State Park, among other places, put the "gold" in South Carolina's Golden Corner.

GPS COORDINATES

UTM Zone (WGS84) 17S

Easting 0307340

Northing 3858700

Latitude 34 51' 44.7"

Longitude 83 6' 6.2"

TABLE ROCK STATE PARK

THE DISTINCTIVE GRANITE FACE of Table Rock Mountain has attracted people to this scenic area since the days of the Cherokee, who believed the Great Spirit dined on the mountain's flat top, hence the name Table Rock. Later, this area was developed by the Civilian Conservation Corps during the Great Depression. The Corps' handiwork was so well crafted that Table Rock Mountain State Park was placed on the National Register of Historic Places in 1989.

Not that this park needed man's imprint to be special. Waterfalls, deep forests, and rock outcrops adorned the mountains long before the 3,083 acres became a state park in 1935. The facilities just make it more user-friendly.

The campground suffices for the tent camper who likes to be on the move, but it's not an end in itself. The main camping area has 75 sites spread on a two-loop setup in open, rolling woods that have suffered the ravages of many storms, which made pulp of the pine trees that once dotted the campground. In addition, little is left of the understory, minimizing privacy. It's strange to see a campground with electrical and water hookups at each site but no elaborate site shaping or defined tent pads. But don't let that scare you—only 20 of the sites are designated as pull-throughs, which translates to RVs. The six primitive walk-in sites offer seclusion and value for tent campers.

The first eight sites lie along the approach road and are very open. Unless you have visited before, you won't have a favorite site to reserve, but don't let that deter you from coming.

Campsites are placed fairly close together inside the loop. Three bathhouses with flush toilets and hot showers are evenly dispersed among the sites, the exception being the sites on the approach road. Degrees of sun, shade, and slope vary from site to site. Plenty of

> *The wide variety of attractions at this state park will make your stay worthwhile.*

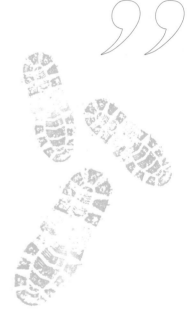

RATINGS

Beauty: ✩ ✩ ✩
Privacy: ✩ ✩ ✩
Spaciousness: ✩ ✩
Quiet: ✩ ✩ ✩
Security: ✩ ✩ ✩ ✩ ✩
Cleanliness: ✩ ✩ ✩ ✩ ✩

ADDRESS: 158 East Ellison Ln. Pickens, SC 29671

OPERATED BY: South Carolina State Parks

INFORMATION: (864) 878-9813; southcarolina parks.com; reservations: (866) 345-7275, reserve america.com

OPEN: Year-round

SITES: 6 walk-in primitive sites, 96 drive-in sites with water and electricity

EACH SITE: Walk-in sites have picnic tables, fire rings, and tent pads; other sites also have water and electricity

ASSIGNMENT: All sites may be reserved

REGISTRATION: At camp store or at Table Rock visitor center

FACILITIES: Water, hot showers, camp store, laundry

PARKING: At campsites only

FEE: $6–$8 walk-in sites, $16–$18 other sites (prices for both vary depending on season)

ELEVATION: 1,160 feet

RESTRICTIONS: *Pets:* On leash only *Fires:* In fire rings only *Alcohol:* Prohibited *Vehicles:* None *Other:* 14-day stay limit

level, shaded sites are available. Expect the best ones to be taken during the weekends.

Located in thicker woods on a dead-end road, the White Oaks Campground area may actually be preferable to the main camping area if you like less hustle and bustle. Its 25 sites are spread along a loop and share a single bathhouse in the loop's center with flush toilets for each sex.

The primitive camping area is on the south side of SC 11, near the visitor center and park office. The sites here are set on a ridge near Lake Oolenoy. Pines shade the sites, which are a 500-plus-foot walk. Site 1 is on a slope, but 2 is set above it. Sites 3 and 4 are together and are the best shaded. Sites 5 and 6 are highest on the hill. Water and a pit toilet are located on a trail near the six sites.

At Table Rock, the campground is just a place to rest and eat between activities. Two lakes lie within the park's confines. Pinnacle Lake finds summertime campers relaxing on its beach or jumping off the high and low diving boards into the clear, cool waters. Canoeists fish for bass, bream, or catfish, and pedal boaters take scenic rides atop the lake's 36 acres.

If water is not your thing, get together with the full-time park naturalist. Many programs are offered during summer. The Table Rock Nature Center has displays that detail the natural history of the region. Children can have fun at the playground.

None of the above would be there if it weren't for the natural beauty of Table Rock. And the best way to enjoy these South Carolina mountain lands is on foot. A 10-mile trail network emanates from the nature center. The 3.4-mile Table Rock Trail lives up to its national recreation trail status. It leads upward among giant boulders to Pinnacle Ridge at Panther Gap. From Panther Gap, the trail climbs the steps of Governor's Rock (which offers a view) to reach the top of Table Rock at 3 miles. Hike another half mile to enjoy a more views of the South Carolina countryside.

Pinnacle Mountain Trail is very challenging. It passes Mill Creek Falls and Bald Rock on the way to the 3,425-foot peak, the park's highest point. A 2-mile connector trail links Pinnacle Mountain and Table

MAP

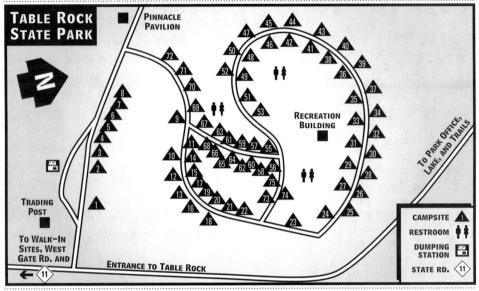

TABLE ROCK STATE PARK

PINNACLE PAVILION

RECREATION BUILDING

TO PARK OFFICE, LAKE, AND TRAILS

TRADING POST

TO WALK-IN SITES, WEST GATE RD. AND

ENTRANCE TO TABLE ROCK

← 11

CAMPSITE ▲
RESTROOM 👫
DUMPING STATION
STATE RD. ◇11

Rock trails. Carrick Creek Nature Trail offers a shorter 1.8-mile loop through forest characteristic of this worthwhile park. Every path here is a winner.

GETTING THERE

From Pickens drive north on US 178 9 miles. Turn right on SC 11, and follow it 4.4 miles to West Gate Road. The park is a half mile up West Gate Road.

GPS COORDINATES

UTM Zone (WGS84) 17S
Easting 0344570
Northing 3877120
Latitude 35 1' 35.3"
Longitude 82 42' 13.0"

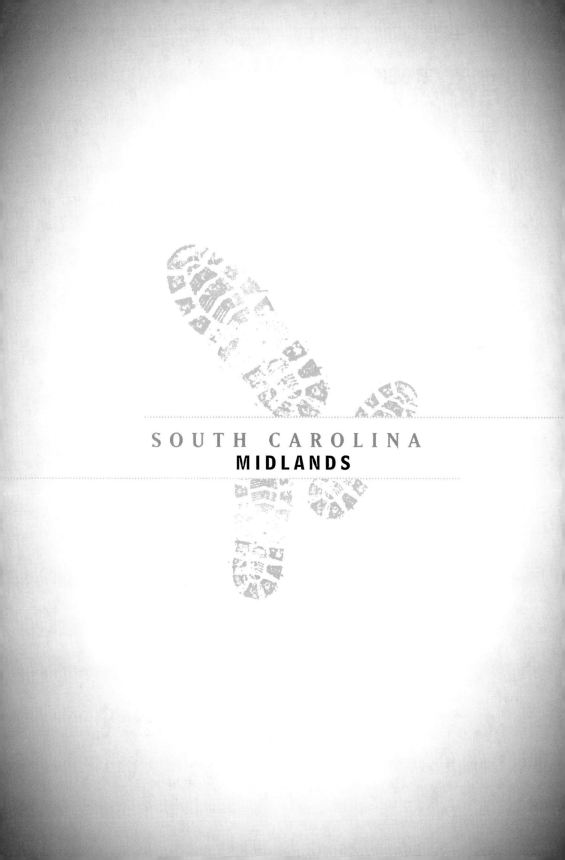

SOUTH CAROLINA
MIDLANDS

T WAS A GORGEOUS SPRING AFTERNOON when I arrived at Baker Creek State Park. The yellow sun was glinting through the spring-green trees. Lake Thurmond, or Lake J. Strom Thurmond as it is formally known, was rippling as I rolled through the hills of the well-manicured park. Birds were singing the praises of rebirth. I found the camping area and turned into camping Loop 1. The hillside and lakefront camps were inviting—yet there wasn't a soul in them! I couldn't understand why and sought out the park manager, who explained that the electricity had been taken out of the loop; therefore, the electric loop, Loop 2, got most of the business. From my point of view, Loop 1 has been improved with no electricity, and it is only a matter of time before the word spreads that a tent-only loop with lakefront campsites is available.

RVs are prohibited in Loop 1, which is actually a loop within a loop. It is set on a peninsula jutting into Lake Thurmond. Pines, oaks, hickories, and sweetgum trees shade the campsites here; dogwoods and cedars compose the understory. Higher on the hill, the inner loop has sites 1 through 24, which afford a commanding view of the lake below. The lower loop, with sites 24 through 50, offers lakefront camping, where you can pull your boat up or swim at the campsite. The red-clay camping pads are a little on the small side, and vegetation between sites is limited. But privacy isn't much of an issue here, as you are unlikely to have a neighbor, and if you do, there is a site far enough away for you to obtain the privacy you want. Depending on where you are, you can either face out to the main lake or into coves on either side of the peninsula. Two bathhouses, a bit antiquated, serve the loop.

Loop 2, with electricity, is popular with the RV set and can be more crowded. The 50-site camping area is set on the next peninsula over, jutting into the

> *The lakefront sites on the tent-camping loop are nearly always available.*

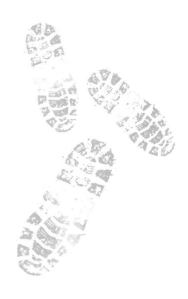

RATINGS

Beauty: ✩ ✩ ✩
Privacy: ✩ ✩ ✩ ✩
Spaciousness: ✩ ✩ ✩
Quiet: ✩ ✩ ✩
Security: ✩ ✩ ✩ ✩
Cleanliness: ✩ ✩ ✩ ✩

ADDRESS: 863 Baker Creek Rd. McCormick, SC 29835

OPERATED BY: South Carolina State Parks

INFORMATION: (864) 443-2457; southcarolina parks.com; reservations: (866) 345-7275, reserve america.com

OPEN: Loop 1, March 1– September 30; Loop 2, year-round

SITES: 50 tent-only sites, 50 others

EACH SITE: Picnic table, water spigot; some sites have upright grills; Loop 2 also has electricity

ASSIGNMENT: First come, first served and by reservation

REGISTRATION: At park office

FACILITIES: Hot showers, flush toilets

PARKING: At campsites only

FEE: $10–$14 tent sites, $15–$18 electric sites (prices for both vary depending on season)

ELEVATION: 350 feet

RESTRICTIONS: *Pets:* On leash only *Fires:* In fire rings only *Alcohol:* Prohibited *Vehicles:* No RVs in tent-camping area *Other:* 14-day stay limit

lake. It also has two bathhouses. There is no need to stay in this crowded area when you will likely have but one or two neighbors in Loop 1. (By the way, if Loop 1 is closed, just find the park manager and he will open it for you.)

Part of the allure of Baker Creek is the park staff. They offer friendliness with every visit; some of the larger Army Corps of Engineers parks on the lake can't offer that. The state park is a water-oriented destination, as it is on the shores of Lake Thurmond. Anglers vie for bass, crappie, and catfish. Two boat ramps are here as well. Swimming is a popular pastime; you can do so at your campsite or near the park office, but no lifeguards are provided. A shaded pavilion overlooks the lake near the park office. The park also has a 10-mile mountain-bike trail that draws visitors in, especially in spring and fall. This trail is part of a greater network of mountain-bike trails in this part of South Carolina. Nearby Hickory Knob State Park, also in McCormick County, has 12 miles of trails open to mountain bikers. Hikers have two short nature trails to walk at Baker Creek.

The whole park slows down in summer, as it is excessively hot. April and May are the best months to visit, followed by September and October. The gate is locked at night for your safety, and rangers reside on-site. If you forgot something, the nearby town of McCormick has a full-service grocery store.

MAP

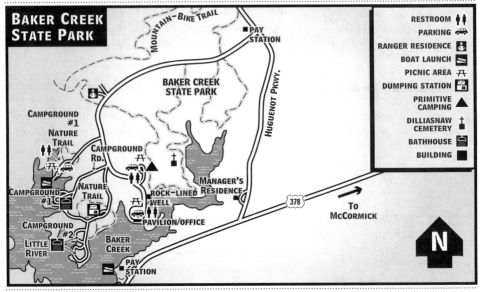

BAKER CREEK STATE PARK

MOUNTAIN-BIKE TRAIL

BAKER CREEK STATE PARK

HUGUENOT PKWY.

CAMPGROUND #1

NATURE TRAIL

CAMPGROUND Rd.

CAMPGROUND #1

NATURE TRAIL

CAMPGROUND #2

LITTLE RIVER

BAKER CREEK

ROCK-LINED WELL

PAVILION/OFFICE

MANAGER'S RESIDENCE

PAY STATION

PAY STATION

378

To McCormick

N

	RESTROOM
	PARKING
	RANGER RESIDENCE
	BOAT LAUNCH
	PICNIC AREA
	DUMPING STATION
	PRIMITIVE CAMPING
	DILLIASNAW CEMETERY
	BATHHOUSE
	BUILDING

GETTING THERE

From McCormick, take US 378 west 3.7 miles to a right turn on Huguenot Parkway. Turn right on Huguenot Parkway, and follow it 1.1 miles to the state park entrance, on your left.

GPS COORDINATES

UTM Zone (WGS84) 17S

Easting 0371560

Northing 3751940

Latitude 33 53' 0.6"

Longitude 82 21' 31.4"

> *This quiet campground is a base for those traveling the Buncombe Trail.*

TALK ABOUT TRANSITION—one minute I was zipping along I-26, and the next I was at Brick House Campground. The place was so quiet that I could hear myself breathe. Rushing down the interstate was exactly what I was trying to get away from. The serene atmosphere and quaint natural setting of Brick House were exactly what tent campers want. Brick House delivered, so much so that I just hung around the campsite all day reveling in the clear, crisp fall air that had swept over the South Carolina Midlands. The next day I hiked the nearby Buncombe Trail. A mountain bike would've been an even better means of traveling this trail, but I was regrettably bikeless. However, mountain bikers are discovering and enjoying this path in ever-increasing numbers.

The Enoree District of the Sumter National Forest is just a short drive up I-26 from Columbia. So it makes sense that the Buncombe Trail is catching on. But the lack of use at Brick House Campground is surprising. Sure, a few equestrians, hunters, and family campers find their way here, but this place can be a nice base camp for trail enthusiasts, too. Despite being only 4 miles from the interstate, Brick House seems a world away.

After passing the Buncombe Trailhead, enter the campground loop, where tall pines form the forest superstory. Elms, dogwoods, sweetgums, and other hardwoods grow beneath the taller evergreens. The forest floor is littered with pine needles and pointy sweetgum balls.

There is little brush between campsites, but privacy isn't as much of an issue as you would think. Because this campground rarely, if ever, fills, you likely won't have a neighbor next to you. Sites 1 and 2 are close together and act as a double site. The woods are sparse behind these camps due to cutting from a pine-beetle infestation, but most pines in the campground loop have been spared. The water spigot has been

RATINGS

Beauty: ☆ ☆ ☆
Privacy: ☆ ☆
Spaciousness: ☆ ☆ ☆ ☆
Quiet: ☆ ☆ ☆ ☆
Security: ☆ ☆ ☆
Cleanliness: ☆ ☆ ☆

dismantled, so bring your own water. Come to large, open sites on the outside of the loop. A stone marker for the Youth Conservation Corps, which rehabilitated this campground and Buncombe Trail, is next to the road. Site 12 is purely in pines. Curve around to reach the shady sites.

Notice the white-banded trees near some sites. These are where occasional horse campers can tie their animals. The terrain slopes away from the campground as the loop turns back toward Brick House Road. Some open sites lie on the inside of the loop. Come to a group of three shady sites at the campground's end. This is where I stayed, in 23. Two "sweet-smelling-technology" vault toilets serve the campground.

You may notice blue blazes on trees running behind site 13. This is the Buncombe Trail. You can pick it up there or start at the trailhead, located just a short piece down Brick House Road, which you passed on the way in. The Buncombe Trail, open to hikers, bikers, and equestrians, is broken into colored segments of different lengths. It circles the Headley Creek watershed through environments typical of the Piedmont. The Red Trail cuts across the main loop, allowing two loop trips of 9 and 12 miles, respectively. Hikers, mountain bikers, and equestrians are welcome to enjoy this trail. Trail maps are posted at signboards in the campground and at the trailhead. South Carolina's master path, Palmetto Trail, runs in conjunction with part of Buncombe Trail. I've hiked nearly the entire trail system. Bring your hiking boots and a two-wheeler to double your fun at this first-rate spring and fall Midlands destination. It's a regular stop in my Palmetto wanderings.

KEY INFORMATION

ADDRESS:	20 Work Center Rd. Whitmire, SC 29178
OPERATED BY:	U.S. Forest Service
INFORMATION:	(864) 427-9858; fs.fed.us/r8/fms
OPEN:	Year-round
SITES:	23
EACH SITE:	Picnic table, fire ring; most sites also have lantern posts
ASSIGNMENT:	First come, first served; no reservations
REGISTRATION:	Self-registration on site
FACILITIES:	Vault toilets
PARKING:	At campsites only
FEE:	$5
ELEVATION:	450 feet
RESTRICTIONS:	*Pets:* On leash only *Fires:* In fire rings only *Alcohol:* At campsites only *Vehicles:* No more than two per site *Other:* 14-day stay limit

MAP

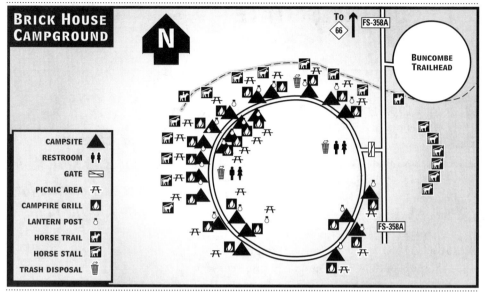

GETTING THERE

From Exit 60 on I-26 near Clinton, take SC 66 east 3.6 miles to Brick House Road. Turn right on Brick House Road, Forest Service Road 358, and follow it 0.5 miles to reach the campground, on your right.

GPS COORDINATES

UTM Zone (WGS84) 17S
Easting 0435020
Northing 3811540
Latitude 34 26' 43.0"
Longitude 81 42' 25.6"

DON'T LOOK FOR SOME BIG WATERFALL when you come to this lakeside recreation area. Before the damming of Richard B. Russell Lake, the Savannah River once flowed free. At high water, a rapid on the Savannah River, near where the Calhoun family resided, resembled a waterfall. Now, Calhoun Falls is just the name of a town and a nearby state recreation area centered on large Lake Richard B. Russell. The U.S. Army Corps of Engineers developed this impoundment, the middle of three consecutive large reservoirs damming the Savannah River. Part of the Corps' work was on Calhoun Falls State Recreation Area, which it turned over to the South Carolina state park system to manage. The walk-in tent sites here should serve as models for other parks to follow.

Good campsites are expensive to build, and the Corps of Engineers spared no expense here. This is evident in the fixtures of every campsite you see, with first-rate fire grates, picnic tables, lantern posts, and more. The walk-in tent sites are near Campground 2. The first set of walk-in sites comprises T-5 through T-0 (you reach the sites in reverse order). Dip into thick woods and a streamside hollow. T-5 is in a flat beside the hollow. Landscaping timbers have been laid into the hillside to level the campsites, which have a sand floor. Cross two footbridges to reach T-4, which is very shady and has a walkway to the lake. The path leaves the hollow and reaches sites overlooking an arm of the lake. T-3 is more open but is shaded by water oak, cedar, and a few other trees. Bring a canopy during midsummer for sun protection. T-2 directly overlooks the water. T-1 is set on a point; shade is limited, but the water panorama is appealing. T-0, over a hill, offers maximum solitude. The walk from the parking area to T-0 is about 140 yards.

> *The awesome walk-in tent sites here should serve as models for other parks to follow.*

RATINGS

Beauty: ✿ ✿ ✿ ✿
Privacy: ✿ ✿ ✿ ✿
Spaciousness: ✿ ✿ ✿ ✿ ✿
Quiet: ✿ ✿ ✿ ✿
Security: ✿ ✿ ✿ ✿ ✿
Cleanliness: ✿ ✿ ✿

ADDRESS: 46 Maintenance
Park Rd.
Calhoun Falls, SC
29628

OPERATED BY: South Carolina
State Parks

INFORMATION: (864) 447-8267;
southcarolina
parks.com;
reservations:
(866) 345-7275,
reserve
america.com

OPEN: Year-round

SITES: 14 walk-in tent
sites, 86 others

EACH SITE: Walk-in sites have
picnic tables, fire
rings, lantern
posts, cooking
tables; other sites
also have water
and electricity

ASSIGNMENT: First come, first
served and by
reservation

REGISTRATION: At tackle shop

FACILITIES: Hot showers, flush
toilets, vault toi-
lets, water spigots

PARKING: At walk-in-camper
parking area and
at campsites

FEE: $14–$16 walk-in
sites, $19–$22
other sites,
depending on
season

ELEVATION: 500 feet

RESTRICTIONS: *Pets:* On leash only
Fires: In fire rings
only
Alcohol: Prohibited
Vehicles: No more
than two per site
Other: 14-day stay
limit

The second walk-in area is home to sites T-6 through T-13, located on the upper end of a cove. T-6 and T-7 are so close to the parking area as to almost lose their walk-in status. That is not to say they are bad—they aren't. The camps are directly on the water. T-8 and T-9 are also on the water but are more shaded. T-10 has easy access to the parking area but not to the lake. T-11 is thickly shaded but is off the lake. Cross footbridges to reach T-12. Shaded and on the water, it is highly recommended. T-13, another shady site, is the farthest from the parking area. A path from T-13 leads to the water. All sites here, including the walk-in tent sites, are reservable. Oddly, the walk-in sites generally fill only on holiday weekends. An outdoor shower, water spigots, and vault toilets are in the immediate campground vicinity. Tent campers can use the show-ers at the other campgrounds.

Two other large campgrounds, Campground 1 and Campground 2, serve the park. They are leveled, landscaped, and well thought out, mixing pull-through sites with pull-up sites for RVs and tent campers who wish to have on-site water and electricity. A look at these two lakeside camping areas shows that no expense was spared here either. Campground 1 is closed during the off-season.

The developed recreation areas are nice, too. The beach house for the lake's swim area is beyond elabo-rate for a park structure. Tennis courts and a basketball court are located near the beach house. Cedar Bluff Nature Trail leaves from near the beach house and makes a 1.75-mile loop.

Most of the other recreation opportunities center on Lake Russell (named after a Georgia politician to offset the naming of another lake downstream for the venerable U.S. Sen. J. Strom Thurmond from South Carolina). The recreation area has its own marina, boat ramp, dock, and tackle shop. The Savannah River forms much of the border between South Carolina and Georgia. Lake Russell covers 26,000 acres, plenty of room to enjoy the water sport of your choice. If you don't have a boat, you can cast your line from one of the two park fishing piers. One is located near the walk-in area by site 56 of Campground 2. The other pier is

MAP

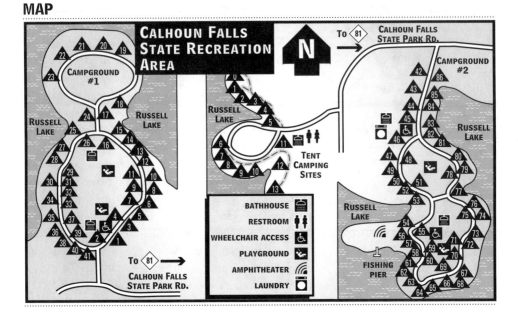

by the boat ramp. Just remember that one water feature you won't see at this fine destination is a waterfall.

GETTING THERE

From Abbeville, take SC 72 west 15 miles to the town of Calhoun Falls and SC 81. Turn right on SC 81, and follow it 1.1 miles to the state recreation area, on your left.

GPS COORDINATES

UTM Zone (WGS84) 17S
Easting 0350920
Northing 3775030
Latitude 34 6' 25.8"
Longitude 82 36' 59.1"

> " *This large state park complements an adjacent Revolutionary War battlefield.* "

DID YOU KNOW THAT MORE Revolutionary War battles took place in South Carolina than in any other state? Take the Battle of Kings Mountain, which took place on October 7, 1780, and is considered the turning point for the Americans in the South. Frontiersmen from North Carolina, South Carolina, Tennessee, and Virginia gathered to defeat Lord Cornwallis and end the British advance into North Carolina. The Loyalists and English army were forced to retreat back to Charleston, ultimately to lose the war. Today, you can visit this battlefield, known as Kings Mountain National Military Park, and pitch your tent at the adjacent Kings Mountain State Park, which functions as the recreational counterpart to the battlefield. Here, you can hike, swim, fish, and enjoy yet more American history beyond the battlefield.

Campsites at the state park are widespread among pines and oaks. As you pass the Trading Post, a small campground store, the ridgetop camping area slopes away from the main campsites. The first large loop has 75 sites, which are shared by tent campers, pop-ups, and RVs. The second major loop has the balance of the sites, including walk-in tent sites. The tent campers' parking area is near site 82. Beyond the parking area and along the loop, sites are far enough in the woods to lend a rustic atmosphere, but not so far back that you'll feel like a mine mule after setting up camp. The understory is much thicker among the tent sites, with brush and smaller trees complementing the shady forest. Descend along a ridgeline between two narrow hollows to find site T-1, which is closest to the parking area. T-2 and T-3 are next to a dry streambed. A trail leads past T-4. As the loop begins to curve back uphill, reach T-5, which is a bit sloped. T-6, set among many pines, has a water spigot near it. I would be proud to pitch my tent at T-7 or T-8. The loop curves back toward the parking

RATINGS

Beauty: ☆ ☆ ☆
Privacy: ☆ ☆ ☆
Spaciousness: ☆ ☆ ☆ ☆
Quiet: ☆ ☆ ☆
Security: ☆ ☆ ☆ ☆ ☆
Cleanliness: ☆ ☆ ☆ ☆

area, making sites T-9 and T-10 easily accessible.

A campground host assists campers during the warmer months. Numerous bathhouses are evenly spread among the loops, including one near the tent campers' parking area. A recreation building at the campground makes rainy days more livable. The campground sees the most traffic during spring and fall but only fills on major summer holidays and Pioneer Days in September. Pioneer Days is a festival centered on a historic homestead at the state park that replicates an 1840s farm. Highlights include crafts, music, and a muzzle-loader-shooting competition. A trail connects the campground to the living-history farm. The campground also sees some traffic from I-85 travelers, but walk-in tent campers can nearly always get a site.

The state park offers 7,000 acres, which, combined with the 3,000 acres of the military park, make for a lot of roaming space in the shadow of Charlotte. Two lakes add to the attractive park terrain. Lake Crawford covers 15 acres and has a swimming area for hot days. Lake York is larger at 65 acres and offers johnboats for rent, so anglers can vie for bass and bream. Basketball and volleyball courts and a mini-golf course are near the campground.

I really enjoyed the hiking trail that connects the state park to the military park. The path makes a 16-mile loop and has backcountry campsites amid its ridges and bottomlands, where clear streams flow. I have made this loop in a day. Though rewarding it will challenge you. You can bite off bits and pieces of the trail as there are multiple auto-accessible trailheads. If you don't feel like walking to the nearby Kings Mountain battlefield, just make a stop at the visitor center to check out the museum and a film explaining the battle. Then take the 1.5-mile, self-guided loop trail around the battlefield and appreciate one of South Carolina's many Revolutionary War sites.

KEY INFORMATION

ADDRESS:	1277 Park Rd. Blacksburg, SC 29702
OPERATED BY:	South Carolina State Parks
INFORMATION:	(803) 222-3209; southcarolina parks.com, reservations: (866) 345-7275, reserve america.com
OPEN:	Year-round
SITES:	10 walk-in tent sites, 116 others
EACH SITE:	Walk-in sites have picnic tables, tent pads, fire rings; other sites also have water and electricity but no tent pads
ASSIGNMENT:	First come, first served and by reservation
REGISTRATION:	At campground Trading Post April–October; ranger will come by to register you rest of year
FACILITIES:	Hot showers, flush toilets, laundry
PARKING:	At walk-in tent parking and at campsites
FEE:	$12–$13 walk-in tent sites, $16–$18 other sites
ELEVATION:	750 feet
RESTRICTIONS:	*Pets:* On leash only *Fires:* In fire rings only *Alcohol:* Prohibited *Vehicles:* No more than 2 per site *Other:* 14-day stay limit

MAP

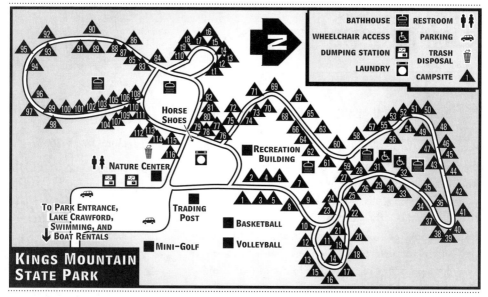

GETTING THERE

From Exit 8/Kings Mountain, on I-85 just north of the North Carolina–South Carolina border, take NC 161 south 5 miles, leaving North Carolina en route. Turn right on Park Road, and follow it into the state park.

GPS COORDINATES

UTM Zone (WGS84) 17S
Easting 0469060
Northing 3889390
Latitude 35 7' 57.5"
Longitude 81 20' 46.0"

LEROY'S FERRY CAMPGROUND

McCormick

THE SHORES OF LAKE THURMOND abound with campgrounds. While scouring them for this book, I found that most were just too big and overly developed. But on arriving at Leroy's Ferry, I knew it was a winner. It was small, primitive, and quiet compared with other campgrounds. The ones that didn't make the cut resembled campground cities, strung out along the shore with signs pointing me here, there, and everywhere while I searched for good sites. I even got lost in the campground of one unmentioned state park along the lake. After that experience, small Leroy's Ferry seemed like home. Its simplicity was a relief.

Simple is the watchword here. This Army Corps of Engineers campground is more about what it doesn't have than what it does have. For starters, it doesn't have a ranger station, confusing signs, hordes of bustling campers, or cars and trailers constantly coming and going. Furthermore, it doesn't have much to do in the way of organized recreation. There are no trails to hike or bike, no nature centers, no boats to rent, no piers from which to fish. The only amenity, in addition to the campground, is a boat launch. You have two choices here: make your own fun on Lake Thurmond or just relax at the campground, which is a fine thing in itself. And for six bucks a day, the price is right. Making your own fun could also include bank fishing or swimming on the shoreline.

Just because this campground is primitive doesn't mean that it's not well kept. The Army Corps of Engineers generally takes good care of its property, which ultimately belongs to us. Reach the end of the dead-end road, and pass the fee station that is near the pump well. A gravel road leads right a quarter-mile to campsites 4 through 1 (you reach the sites in reverse order). The hillside slopes toward the lake, but the sites are

> *This is the most primitive campground on the shores of Lake Thurmond.*

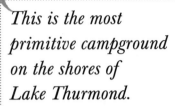

RATINGS

Beauty: ✪ ✪ ✪
Privacy: ✪ ✪ ✪ ✪ ✪
Spaciousness: ✪ ✪ ✪ ✪
Quiet: ✪ ✪ ✪
Security: ✪ ✪ ✪
Cleanliness: ✪ ✪ ✪

ADDRESS: Route 1, Box 6
Clarks Hill, SC
29821

OPERATED BY: U.S. Army Corps
of Engineers

INFORMATION: (800) 533-3478;
sas.usace.army.
mil/lakes/
thurmond

OPEN: Year-round

SITES: 10

EACH SITE: Picnic table, fire
grate, lantern
post; most sites
have upright grills

ASSIGNMENT: First come,
first served;
no reservations

REGISTRATION: Self-registration
on site

FACILITIES: Pump well, vault
toilets

PARKING: At campsites only

FEE: $6

ELEVATION: 340 feet

RESTRICTIONS: *Pets:* On leash only
Fires: In fire rings
only
Alcohol: At camp-
sites only
Vehicles: None
Other: 14-day stay
limit

mostly level. Site 4 is large and overlooks the lake. Site 3 is a good distance away in thick woods. Pine grows highest above these sites, followed by a thick bank of winged elm, sweetgum, and oak. Smaller trees and brush create more than ample privacy. Site 2 is less shady. Site 1 is close to the lake.

Return to the main road that shortly splits. The paved road leading left dead-ends at the boat ramp. A second gravel road that splits right has sites 10 through 5. Site 10 is large and closest to the boat ramp. Site 9 is well above the lake, while sites 8 and 7 are separated by thick woods yet are open toward Lake Thurmond. I stayed in site 6 because it provided good afternoon shade on a hot summer day. Site 5 is at the road's end. Informal trails lead a short distance from these sites to the lake. Despite having only 10 sites, the campground fills only on holiday weekends. Other than then, you should get a site.

People come here for water recreation, whether it be fishing, boating, skiing, or swimming. And Lake Thurmond is a huge recreation destination. Completed in 1954, the lake now hosts 7 million visitors annually. But it doesn't seem that way at Leroy's Ferry. After all, a tent camper can still find a little solitude along the 1,200 miles of shoreline here. Plus, more than 100 islands add a scenic touch to the impoundment. It seems the lake also has 100 campgrounds, but you will likely find that the few sites at Leroy's Ferry offer the best in tent camping.

MAP

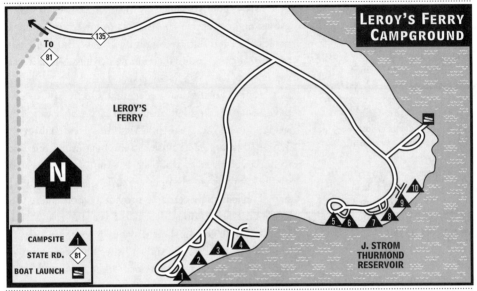

LEROY'S FERRY CAMPGROUND

LEROY'S FERRY

To 81

N

135

J. STROM THURMOND RESERVOIR

CAMPSITE
STATE RD. 81
BOAT LAUNCH

GPS COORDINATES

UTM Zone (WGS84) 17S

Easting 0362180

Northing 3754300

Latitude 33 55' 19.6"

Longitude 82 29' 27.1"

GETTING THERE

From McCormick, take
SC 28 north 7 miles to
SC 81, and veer left, staying
with SC 81 north 5.5 miles to
the hamlet of Wilmington.
Turn left at the signed turn
for Leroy's Ferry Camp-
ground, going just a few feet
over defunct railroad tracks;
then immediately turn right
onto SC 196. Follow SC 196
0.5 miles; then turn left
on SC 135, and follow it
4 miles to dead-end
at the campground.

> *This little valley campground seems a world away from the surrounding area.*

CAMPGROUNDS AND RECREATION AREAS with lakes come in all sizes. Lick Fork Lake is a mere 12 acres, small compared with most impoundments, especially compared with nearby Lake Thurmond. Lick Fork Lake Campground has only 10 sites—just about the right number to handle this lake. Located in the surprisingly deep and secluded valley of Lick Fork (but only 10 miles from a town), the area exudes a close, intimate feel, as if you are in the middle of nowhere. The no-gas-motors rule on the lake, along with the widespread campsites, means that chirping birds and maybe some kids swimming in the clear water will be your only background noise.

I really like this campground. The sites are spacious and spread out far from one another. They are incorporated into a hilly setting with some leveling and stonework that make the sites both attractive and "campable." Oaks and pines provide the shade. A gravel road dips toward Lick Fork Lake, passing a water spigot to reach sites 1 and 2. These are on mostly level terrain. Sand has been spread in individual camping areas, each with a separate tent pad. Sites 3 through 5 are built into a slope. Landscaping stones held together with concrete form leveling walls, resulting in two-tiered sites. As the gravel road curves toward the lake, reach site 6, which overlooks the lake from across the road. Then come to the most favored sites, 7 through 9. These directly overlook Lick Fork Lake, which is just a short down-slope walk away. Site 9 is on a point just above the lake's fishing pier. The road then curves away from the lake into a hollow. The final site here, 10, is usually occupied by the campground host.

The campground, with so much area for so few sites, has four vault toilets. The small number of sites means that it fills quickly at times, especially on weekends during late spring and early summer. Then the

RATINGS

Beauty: ✿ ✿ ✿ ✿
Privacy: ✿ ✿ ✿
Spaciousness: ✿ ✿ ✿
Quiet: ✿ ✿ ✿ ✿
Security: ✿ ✿ ✿ ✿
Cleanliness: ✿ ✿ ✿

heat kicks in and business dies down. Sites are available during the week any time of year. A campground host is on duty most of the warm season and locks the campground gate at 10 p.m., a plus for camper security.

A restroom with cold showers overlooks the swim and picnic area. The picnic shelter here is a nice place to hang out during a summertime thunderstorm. Elaborate stonework has leveled parts of the picnic area, which overlooks a grassy lawn adjacent to the roped-off swim area. The latter has a sandy bottom for cleanfooted entry into and exit out of the pretty lake. A paved walkway with a quaint bridge connects the picnic area to a small fishing pier and the boat launch (as previously mentioned, no gas motors are allowed here). Anglers vie primarily for catfish but also largemouth bass and bream. The clear water and deep valley remind me of a small mountain lake rather than a lake in the South Carolina Midlands.

Two trails emanate from the boat-launch area. The Lick Fork Trail circles around the lake, making a 2-mile circuit that emerges from the woods near the swim area. The Horn Creek Trail is longer, at 5.7 miles. Mountain bikers really enjoy this route, though it sees its share of hikers as well. The path leaves the Lick Fork drainage, then climbs over a ridge to dip into the Horn Creek drainage. From here, the path winds along Horn Creek before returning. It crosses forest roads three times, helping you track your progress. And Horn Creek may be about as far away as you want to get from this hideaway, tucked in the little valley of Lick Fork.

KEY INFORMATION

ADDRESS:	c/o Long Cane Ranger District 810 Buncombe St. Edgefield, SC 29824
OPERATED BY:	Sumter National Forest
INFORMATION:	(803) 637-5396; fs.fed.us/r8/fms
OPEN:	Year-round
SITES:	10
EACH SITE:	Picnic table, fire ring, tent pad
ASSIGNMENT:	First come, first served; no reservations
REGISTRATION:	Self-registration on site
FACILITIES:	Cold showers, flush toilets, vault toilets, water spigots
PARKING:	At campsites only
FEE:	$7
ELEVATION:	350 feet
RESTRICTIONS:	*Pets:* On leash only *Fires:* In fire rings only *Alcohol:* At campsites only *Vehicles:* None *Other:* 14-day stay limit

MAP

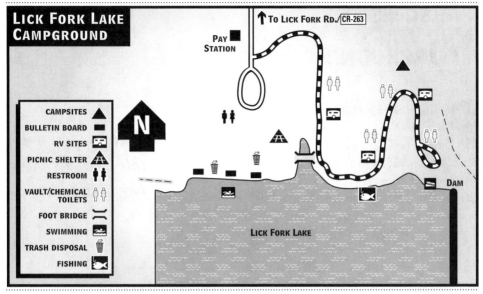

GETTING THERE

From the Edgefield town square, head west on SC 23 8.3 miles to SC 230, Martin-town Road. Veer left on SC 230, and follow it 0.4 miles to CR 263, Lick Fork Road. Turn left on Lick Fork Road, and follow it 2 miles to the campground, on your right.

GPS COORDINATES

UTM Zone (WGS84) 17S
Easting 0403570
Northing 3732450
Latitude 33 43' 45.6"
Longitude 82 2' 26.6"

49
PARSON'S
MOUNTAIN
CAMPGROUND

PARSON'S MOUNTAIN RECREATION AREA, in
Sumter National Forest, offers boating, swimming, fishing, and hiking, along with an excellent campground in a rustic and well-kept setting. One
goal of the U.S. Forest Service is to manage our
national forests for public recreation. It is for this reason that areas like Parson's Mountain are developed.
Under the multiple-use concept, the Forest Service
also manages lands for watershed protection, timber
harvesting, and wildlife enhancement, among other
things. Tent campers benefit greatly from the recreation component of the multiple-use concept.

The roots of the recreation area were planted
decades ago, when the Civilian Conservation Corps
dammed Mountain Creek and developed the resulting
shoreline, including the campground. The historic part
of the recreation area, stonework and such, was left
intact even after the area was modernized, including
the addition of a bathhouse in the day-use area that
complements the traditional campground, in recent
years. You will pass the day-use area before entering
the campground. Campsites 1 and 3 are on an arm of
Parson's Mountain Lake and are the only lakeside sites
here. Oddly, these sites are lesser used than those in the
main campground. Sweetgum, dogwood, pine, cedar,
and elm compose the forest overhead. Continue beyond
a picnic area to enter the main part of the campground,
on a hillside loop.

Starting with campsite 4, the sites are large. They
are well separated from one another and have ample
young trees between them for privacy. Overhead shade
from taller trees varies with the sites but is adequate at
each camping area. Site 10 is of special note, as it is the
most isolated. Most sites on the loop's outside are set
back in the woods; a bathhouse centers the loop. Site
17 is closest to the bathhouse. A short trail connects the

_Tent campers will love
this excellent national
forest recreation area._

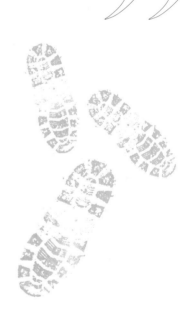

RATINGS

Beauty: ✪ ✪ ✪ ✪
Privacy: ✪ ✪ ✪ ✪
Spaciousness: ✪ ✪ ✪ ✪
Quiet: ✪ ✪ ✪ ✪
Security: ✪ ✪ ✪
Cleanliness: ✪ ✪ ✪

158 **THE BEST IN TENT CAMPING CAROLINAS**

ADDRESS:	c/o Long Cane Ranger District 810 Buncombe St. Edgefield, SC 29824
OPERATED BY:	U.S. Forest Service
INFORMATION:	(803) 637-5396; fs.fed.us/r8/fms
OPEN:	April– mid-December
SITES:	23
EACH SITE:	Picnic table, fire grate, tent pad, lantern post
ASSIGNMENT:	First come, first served; no reservations
REGISTRATION:	Self-registration on site
FACILITIES:	Hot showers, flush toilets, vault toilets, water spigots
PARKING:	At campsites only
FEE:	$7
ELEVATION:	475 feet
RESTRICTIONS:	*Pets:* On leash only *Fires:* In fire rings only *Alcohol:* Prohibited *Vehicles:* No more than two per site *Other:* 14-day stay limit

main loop to the day-use area near site 20. A campground host is on duty during the warm season.

Twenty-three sites is a desirable number for a campground. The size keeps the campground generally quiet, but not so small that it fills too quickly. However, Parson's Mountain does fill on ideal spring and early summer weekends.

At 28 acres, Parson's Mountain Lake is also just the right size. The shoreline is pretty everywhere you look, whether it is the grassy picnic areas shaded by tall pines or the trees growing along the shoreline. No gas motors are allowed, and boaters will be pleased to know that the lake has a boat ramp, making boating or fishing for largemouth bass, bream, and catfish easy. An earthen pier on one side of the lake is where bank fishermen will be found. The primary day-use area has a designated swim beach downhill from the modern bathhouse. This area also has a large picnic shelter, which is a good place to take cover during summer thunderstorms.

The lake is not the only draw here, though. A hiking trail leads from near the lake spillway 1.2 miles to the top of Parson's Mountain, where a fire tower stands. This out-and-back hike has a 400-foot elevation change, a big change in these parts, and offers a varied forestscape along the way. Unfortunately, the fire tower is closed. You can also see evidence of Civil War–era gold mining along the trail. The Parson's Mountain OHV Trail, open to hikers, bikers, and motorized vehicles, makes a 12-mile loop south of the recreation area. It can be accessed by keeping east on Parson's Mountain Road, beyond the turn into the campground to Forest Service Road 515. Turn right on FS 515 to reach the trailhead past the road to the fire tower.

After a visit to Parson's Mountain, you will see that the Forest Service has had great success managing this part of the Sumter National Forest.

MAP

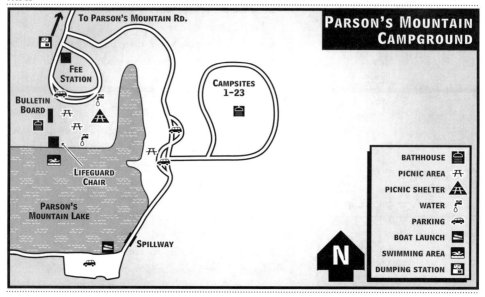

PARSON'S MOUNTAIN CAMPGROUND

To PARSON'S MOUNTAIN RD.

FEE STATION

BULLETIN BOARD

LIFEGUARD CHAIR

PARSON'S MOUNTAIN LAKE

CAMPSITES 1-23

SPILLWAY

BATHHOUSE
PICNIC AREA
PICNIC SHELTER
WATER
PARKING
BOAT LAUNCH
SWIMMING AREA
DUMPING STATION

N

GETTING THERE

From Abbeville, take SC 72 west 2 miles to SC 28. Turn left on SC 28 east, and follow it 2.3 miles to Parson's Mountain Road. Turn left on Parson's Mountain Road, and follow it 1.4 miles to Forest Service Road 514. Turn right on FS 514, and follow it 0.8 miles to reach the campground.

GPS COORDINATES

UTM Zone (WGS84) 17S
Easting 0370620
Northing 3767520
Latitude 34 6' 11.3"
Longitude 82 21' 20.6"

> *This state park is one of South Carolina's most ecologically interesting areas. It has great camping, mountain biking, and hiking, too.*

POINSETT STATE PARK has an interesting location. Set on an outlier of the Carolina Sand Hills, Poinsett is where the vegetation of the low country meets the vegetation of the upcountry, resulting in the overlapping of ecosystems—a place where Spanish moss hangs in trees that stand over blooming mountain-laurel bushes. The melding of nature's finery results in a beautiful setting for a park, and an understanding of why this was an early addition to the South Carolina state park system, originally developed by the Civilian Conservation Corps in the 1930s. Historic structures from the CCC–era add charm to an already pretty place. Another plus in the location department is Poinsett's proximity to Manchester State Forest, which effectively adds thousands of acres to the activity area, where hiking and mountain-biking trails abound. Add a camping loop used exclusively by tent aficionados, and you have a great outdoor destination in the Palmetto State.

The campground is set high on a hill, but the sites, laid out in a classic double loop, are mostly level up here. Pines, oaks, sweetgums, dogwoods, and hickories, draped in Spanish moss, stand over sandy sites. Ample ground vegetation divides the sites and provides good privacy. Two bathhouses serve the locale.

The first loop, the original one, has electric sites. Also note the rock fire rings from the CCC days in the first few sites. The second loop, at the back of the campground, is where tent campers want to be. The loop once had electricity, but it was taken out. However, each site still has its own water spigot. The large, shady sites allow room for all the extras you can cram in your vehicle. A few sites have tent pads, but the sandy floors already make for a level, easy-draining surface. The campground loops around and passes by a large field, then reenters

RATINGS

Beauty: ✰ ✰ ✰ ✰ ✰
Privacy: ✰ ✰ ✰ ✰
Spaciousness: ✰ ✰ ✰
Quiet: ✰ ✰ ✰
Security: ✰ ✰ ✰ ✰
Cleanliness: ✰ ✰ ✰ ✰

the first loop. Note the recreation building here, which could come in handy during rain spells.

Campsites are always available in the nonelectric loop; however, you can make reservations. Once you come here, in fact, you can find the site you like and reserve it for the next trip. Poinsett is a spring and fall destination: summer can be excessively hot, and there is no swimming here. Note that you may experience noise from a nearby bombing range.

The CCC dammed Shanks Creek to create 10-acre Old Levi Mill Lake. The scenic, watery valley offers boating and fishing in a quiet setting where gas motors are not allowed. You can rent a johnboat from the park at a low rate or bring your own canoe, kayak, or other boat, as long as you can carry it to the water, since there is no boat launch. Bass, bream, and catfish lie beneath the placid pond.

Most campers travel the extensive trail system that spreads over the state park and Manchester State Forest. South Carolina's master path, the Palmetto Trail, which extends from the mountains to the sea, heads through here in what is known as the High Hills of Santee Passage. This segment of the Palmetto Trail is 14 miles long from end to end.

The Coquina Trail makes a loop around Old Levi Mill Lake, which connects to another loop trail, the Hilltop Trail, which in turn connects to the Laurel Group Trail. The Equestrian Trail, also open to hikers, makes a 6-mile loop among valleys cut by spring-fed creeks. Swamp vegetation, such as tupelo and cypress, grows next to mountain vegetation, such as galax and mountain laurel, on the hills.

On the way in, you pass the main mountain-biking trailhead for the 25,000-acre Manchester State Forest, which has trails aplenty. Three trails make loops covering more than 17 miles of pedaling. The Killer 3 Trail is the longest, at 10 miles. Be prepared for some of the hilliest terrain in this part of the state and also for sand as you are in the sandhills. Some riding can be quite technical. The trails are open only on Sundays during the fall hunting season, so consider coming in spring for more riding opportunities. Also, a permit is

KEY INFORMATION

ADDRESS:	6660 Poinsett Park Rd. Wedgefield, SC 29168
OPERATED BY:	South Carolina State Parks
INFORMATION:	(803) 494-8177; southcarolina parks.com; reservations: (866) 345-7275, reserve america.com
OPEN:	Year-round
SITES:	25 nonelectric, 25 electric
EACH SITE:	Picnic table, water spigot; some sites have fire rings
ASSIGNMENT:	First come, first served and by reservation
REGISTRATION:	At park office by lake
FACILITIES:	Hot showers, flush toilets
PARKING:	At campsites only
FEE:	$9–$10 per night tent sites, depending on season; $12–$13 per night other sites
ELEVATION:	185 feet
RESTRICTIONS:	*Pets:* On leash only *Fires:* In fire rings only *Alcohol:* Prohibited *Vehicles:* No more than two per site *Other:* No more than six campers per site

MAP

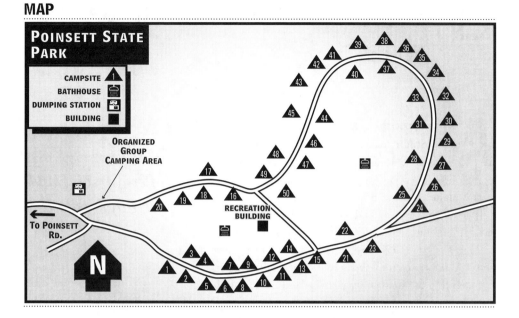

POINSETT STATE PARK

CAMPSITE
BATHHOUSE
DUMPING STATION
BUILDING

ORGANIZED GROUP CAMPING AREA

RECREATION BUILDING

To POINSETT RD.

N

GETTING THERE

From Exit 9 on I-77 in Columbia, take US 378 east, Garners Ferry Road, 26 miles to SC 261. Turn right on SC 261 south, and follow it 10.1 miles, passing through Wedgefield, to reach Poinsett Road. Turn right at the signed turn and follow Poinsett Road 1.7 miles to enter the state park.

required to bike the trails. For information on obtaining one, visit **state.sc.us/forest/permit.htm.** This way, you will be prepared for your visit to Poinsett State Park.

GPS COORDINATES

UTM Zone (WGS84) 17S
Easting 0543190
Northing 3740770
Latitude 33 48' 28.6"
Longitude 80 32' 0.0"

51
SAND HILLS
STATE FOREST

Patrick

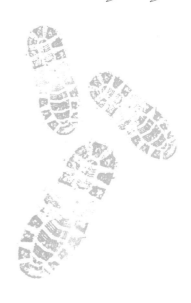

APREHISTORIC SEA ONCE COVERED what is now South Carolina, depositing sand over a wide area. Later, these seas retreated, leaving a region of deep, infertile hills of sand. Over time, many plants and animals adapted to these hills, but settlers farming the land couldn't thrive as nature could. The state eventually acquired the land and now manages 46,000-acre Sand Hills State Forest. Here, tent campers can enjoy the activities of the forest, such as mountain biking, hiking, fishing, and exploring the unique ecosystem.

You get to camp on a hill so big that it's called a mountain—Sugarloaf Mountain. Height is relative here at the edge of the Midlands, but there are scenic views toward the coastal plain in parts of the forest.

Enter the campground via Mountain Road, dipping to Mountain Pond, a small but pretty impoundment of 10 acres. To your right are two large picnic shelters made of wood and stone, flanked by campsites 1-A and 1-B. Campers can use these rustic shelters, which overlook Mountain Pond. Oaks, dogwoods, and pines shade the sites, though the trees are widely separated in the area. Cross over the pond dam. Site 2 has a shelter and also overlooks the lake. Begin to climb Sugarloaf Mountain, passing sites 3 and 4 on the left. Reach the upper end of the mountain, where three more sites with shelters lie between Sugarloaf and Horseshoe mountains. (These so-called mountains are really large hills, which can be climbed via erosion-preventing wooden stairs placed on the hillsides.) Site 7 offers excellent solitude.

The second camping area, with sites 8 through 15, is available for equestrian groups and tent campers. It is more open and sandy. (Be aware that tent campers are encouraged to use the first seven sites rather than the equestrian area.) Sites 8 and 9 are in a loop beside

> *This unusual ecosystem offers camping and recreation galore.*

RATINGS

Beauty: ☆ ☆ ☆
Privacy: ☆ ☆ ☆ ☆
Spaciousness: ☆ ☆ ☆ ☆ ☆
Quiet: ☆ ☆ ☆
Security: ☆ ☆ ☆
Cleanliness: ☆ ☆ ☆

ADDRESS:	P.O. Box 128 Patrick, SC 29584
OPERATED BY:	South Carolina Forestry Commission
INFORMATION:	(843) 498-6478; state.sc.us/forest/ refshill.htm
OPEN:	Year-round
SITES:	15
EACH SITE:	Picnic table, trash barrel; some sites also have covered shelters
ASSIGNMENT:	First come, first served and by reservation
REGISTRATION:	At forest headquarters
FACILITIES:	Vault toilets
PARKING:	At campsites only
FEE:	$10 sites without shelters, $15 sites with shelters
ELEVATION:	325 feet
RESTRICTIONS:	*Pets:* On leash only *Fires:* In fire rings only *Alcohol:* Prohibited *Vehicles:* None *Other:* 14-day stay limit

Mountain Pond. The remaining sites are in a large loop amid sandy pinewoods. All are very large and offer great privacy and more room than anyone would ever need to pitch a tent. The sites with shelters are the most popular. The only other campground amenity is vault toilets, so bring your own water.

Campsites can be reserved, although the campground traditionally fills only on Easter weekend. Spring and fall are the most popular use periods. Note that you need a trail permit from the forest office for mountain biking, but not for hiking. Call ahead and you can have your permit mailed to you, or you can pick it up at the forest headquarters.

Nearly all campers climb Horseshoe and Sugarloaf mountains as a matter of course. Pick up the trailhead of Long Trail, a 1.7-mile nature path, by leaving Mountain Pond and walking toward SC 29, the way you came in. Others will try their luck fishing in Mountain Pond, where bream and bass ply the waters. The state forest has 13 other fishable ponds, but mountain biking is what's really catching on here.

Sand Hills State Forest has established a mountain-biking trail that starts near its headquarters and offers 11 miles of biking over four loops, the largest of which is 6 miles. Screamer, Vista, and Ho Chi Minh Trail are some names that sections of the bike trail have received. Bikers and other visitors can also enjoy the adjacent Carolina Hills National Wildlife Refuge, where 100 miles of gravel roads await. These roads are only occasionally used by park personnel and are "edging toward single-track," according to the park. Hiking and driving trails also await. I enjoyed driving around the state forest. (Truth be known, I got lost trying a shortcut. Get a map at forest headquarters before you explore.) Nonetheless, I was surprised at the views and the attractive nature of this land. It has so much potential, and with a campground like Sugarloaf Mountain, your base camp is set and waiting for you.

MAP

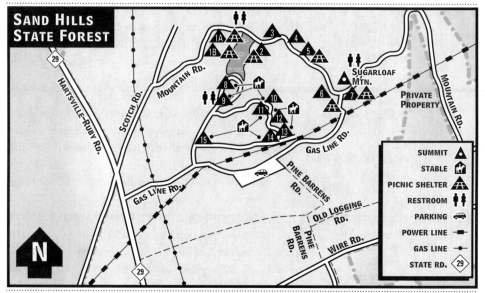

GPS COORDINATES

UTM Zone (WGS84)	17S
Easting	0579480
Northing	3826560
Latitude	34 35' 12.8"
Longitude	80 7' 45.2"

GETTING THERE

From downtown Cheraw, head south on US 1 18 miles to Hartsville–Ruby Road, which is 0.8 miles past the Sand Hill State Forest Headquarters. Turn right on Hartsville–Ruby Road, and follow it 2.8 miles to sandy Forest Service Road 63, Scotch Road. Turn right on Scotch Road, which leaves at an angle, and follow it 0.5 miles. Veer right onto Mountain Road, and reach the camping area with sites 1 through 7. The second area (sites 8 through 15) is off Gas Line Road, leaving SC 29 perpendicular to SC 29, just before Scotch Road.

> *This part of the Sumter National Forest is rich in river recreation.*

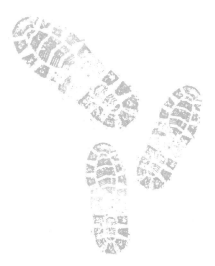

LIKE THE REST OF SOUTH CAROLINA, Woods Ferry Recreation Area is loaded with American history. The adjacent Broad River was an obstacle to travelers of times past. In 1817, Matthew Woods saw an opportunity, acquiring the land that is now the campground and constructing a ferry for people, horses, and buggies to cross the truly broad river. During the Civil War, Confederate General Wade Hampton used the ferry while chasing Union General William Sherman during the latter's infamous March to the Sea, which effectively ended the War between the States. Later, the terrain, like much of the South Carolina Midlands, was logged and then unsoundly farmed, leading to soil erosion. The U.S. Forest Service took over the depleted lands, managing them for timber and recreation. Bridges replaced the ferry both north and south of its former location. Today, Woods Ferry is a rustic recreation area with a quiet campground, hiking, boating, and fishing.

The campground is situated along a sloping valley beside the Broad River. The valley, moister than the area uplands, flourishes in a forest of oaks, elm, and cedars, with a small understory of trees and bushes. Reaching Camping Loop A first, pass the first two sites as the loop angles up the hillside. The sites here are large. Reach a high point at site 10, which is a double. The loop then curves past a bathhouse. The widespread sites don't all have exactly the same amenities, such as lantern posts, because the Forest Service is adding them as funds allow. A factor in picking your site is which particular amenities are available at which sites. The loop flattens out and ends at site 18.

Loop B, which is closer to the Broad River than Loop A, has camping units 19 through 30. Head up a hill, crossing wet-weather streambeds bordered by wood fences, to reach site 22, which is a little open. A

RATINGS

Beauty: ✿ ✿ ✿
Privacy: ✿ ✿ ✿
Spaciousness: ✿ ✿ ✿ ✿
Quiet: ✿ ✿ ✿ ✿
Security: ✿ ✿ ✿
Cleanliness: ✿ ✿ ✿

mini-loop contains the most private sites, including site 29, which is well shaded and close to the day-use area. Each loop has a small bathhouse with hot showers that is walled on the sides but open to the sky. Water spigots are seemingly everywhere in this campground, which rarely, if ever, fills.

Boaters use Woods Ferry occasionally, as do hunters, but overall the place is underused. This is a make-your-own-fun campground. My fun started with the day-use area. Located on a flat beside the Broad River, this area has the right combination of sun, shade, grass, and covered picnic shelters (handy in a rain) for enjoying the Broad River. A boat ramp is used by those with johnboats and canoes floating the Broad. You can put in here and travel 6 or 7 miles downstream to the South Sandy boat ramp. A Forest Service map comes in handy here, so call ahead and order one before your trip. The nearby Tyger and Enoree rivers are excellent for canoeing, with clear water and narrower, more intimate, streamsheds. The Tyger offers 24 miles of floating, while the Enoree offers 36 miles in which you can paddle through the national forest. All three rivers offer freshwater angling.

Also, the Woods Ferry area has a trail system used by hikers, bikers, and horses. It's a little hard to find, so before you take off, check out the trail map on the back of the fee-station signboard. Three loops can be made—3.3, 3.7, and 4 miles—offering forests of the river-floodplain and piedmont types. The first trailhead is about 100 feet behind the fee-station signboard as you face it. The second trail-access point is harder to find—look for the painted blazes on the right side of the day-use area road, a little past the covered signboard in the picnic area. The blazes are on two side-by-side cedar trees. The hand-drawn sketch of the map on the fee-station signboard will help. The map may be rudimentary, but it's a lot easier to get around Woods Ferry today than it was over a hundred years ago, when the ferry was in operation.

KEY INFORMATION

ADDRESS: 3557 Whitmire Hwy. Union, SC 29379

OPERATED BY: U.S. Forest Service

INFORMATION: (864) 427-9858; fs.fed.us/r8/fms

OPEN: Year-round

SITES: 28

EACH SITE: Picnic table, fire ring; some sites also have barbecue pits, upright grills, and/or lantern posts

ASSIGNMENT: First come, first served; no reservations

REGISTRATION: Self-registration on site

FACILITIES: Hot showers, flush toilets, water spigots, vault toilets; showers are shut off November–March

PARKING: At campsites only

FEE: $7

ELEVATION: 400 feet

RESTRICTIONS: *Pets:* On leash only
Fires: In fire rings only
Alcohol: At campsites only
Vehicles: None
Other: 14-day stay limit

MAP

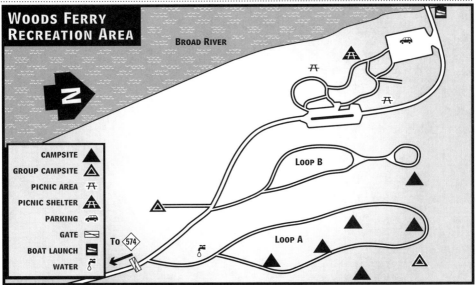

WOODS FERRY RECREATION AREA

BROAD RIVER

LOOP B

LOOP A

To 574

CAMPSITE	▲
GROUP CAMPSITE	△
PICNIC AREA	🏓
PICNIC SHELTER	🏕
PARKING	🚐
GATE	⊠
BOAT LAUNCH	🛥
WATER	💧

GETTING THERE

From Exit 74 on I-26, take SC 34 east 18 miles to SC 215. Turn left on SC 215, and follow it 14.5 miles to SC 72. Turn right on SC 72, and follow it 1.4 miles to SC 25. Turn left on SC 25, Leeds Road, and follow it 2.1 miles; veer left on SC 49, crossing the railroad tracks, and keep on SC 49 3.6 miles to SC 574. Turn left on SC 574, and follow it 3.6 miles to the campground.

GPS COORDINATES

UTM Zone (WGS84) 17S
Easting 0458750
Northing 3839730
Latitude 34 43' 2.7"
Longitude 81 27' 1.4"

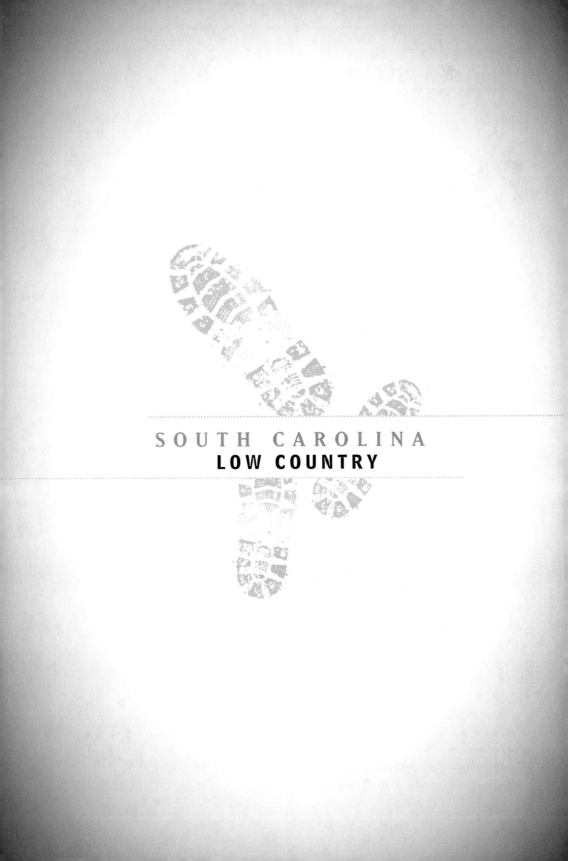

SOUTH CAROLINA
LOW COUNTRY

BEACHFRONT **PROPERTY** is expensive and in high demand these days, making ocean camping a difficult proposition in some places.

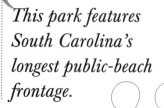

This park features South Carolina's longest public-beach frontage.

Luckily, the state of South Carolina owns 4 miles of beachfront on quiet Hunting Island, overlooking the Atlantic Ocean. Here, tent campers can pitch their shelters in the main campground by the beach or in the seclusion of walk-in tent-camping sites, then explore a restored historic lighthouse and enjoy the natural beauty beyond the beach, where live oak, pine, and palm forests contrast with the grassy estuaries toward the mainland.

Set along the Atlantic shoreline, Hunting Island's widespread campground attracts tent campers with its natural beauty. The first loop has campsites 1 through 59. Live oaks, palms, and slash pines shade these oceanside sites. This is the land of the RVs, but the tent sites are appealing. If you are going to camp here, go for sites 38 through 55, just feet from the beach. The second beachfront loop has sites 60 through 86. These sites are heavily shaded, too, with more pines than live oaks. The best sites here are 61 through 73, carpeted by pine needles, oak leaves, and sand.

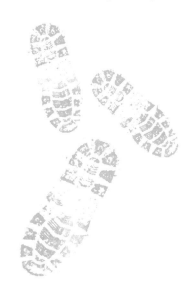

The rear camping area houses sites 89 through 200, laid out in a series of loops. The woods are thicker here, and ancient wooded dunes offer geographic relief to the otherwise flat area. Palmetto and brush add privacy. This rear area also has the two walk-in tent-camping areas, where solitude and quiet reign. The first walk-in area, with sites T-1 through T-5, leaves the main campground near site 162. A sandy path leads to a heavily wooded rolling area, so hilly that tent sites are limited. Some sites have fire grates in addition to picnic tables. The farthest walk is less than 100 yards but seems a world away from the main campground. The second walk-in tent-camping area, near site 177, has sites T-6 through T-10. These are the best tent

RATINGS

Beauty: ☆ ☆ ☆ ☆
Privacy: ☆ ☆ ☆
Spaciousness: ☆ ☆ ☆
Quiet: ☆ ☆ ☆ ☆
Security: ☆ ☆ ☆ ☆ ☆
Cleanliness: ☆ ☆ ☆

KEY INFORMATION

ADDRESS: 2555 Sea Island Pkwy. Hunting Island, SC 29920

OPERATED BY: South Carolina State Parks

INFORMATION: (843) 838-2011; southcarolina parks.com; reservations: (866) 345-7275, reserve america.com

OPEN: Tent sites, April–November; campsites 1–86, year-round

SITES: 10 walk-in tent sites, 180 others

EACH SITE: Tent sites have picnic tables; other sites also have water and electricity

ASSIGNMENT: First come, first served and by reservation

REGISTRATION: At park store

FACILITIES: Hot showers, flush toilet, water spigots

PARKING: At campsites and at walk-in tent-camping parking areas

FEE: $17–$19 walk-in tent sites; $23–$25 other sites, depending on season

ELEVATION: Sea level

RESTRICTIONS: *Pets:* On leash only
Fires: In fire rings only
Alcohol: Prohibited
Vehicles: No more than two per walk-in site
Other: 14-day stay limit

sites, as they are more widespread and larger, and have more level ground among the trees.

A camp store is conveniently located within walking distance of all the sites, and water spigots are located at each walk-in tent area. Eight bathhouses are spread throughout the campground. The walk-in sites fill on holiday weekends but are available any weekday. The rest of the campground fills every weekend during summer and occasionally during the week. Only sites 1 through 40 are reservable. Mosquitoes can be troublesome following rainy periods, so call ahead for the latest bug report.

The beach is what drew me to Hunting Island. I enjoyed walking to the north end of the island, then a good way south, stopping to check out the Hunting Island Lighthouse. Built in 1873, the lighthouse and surrounding grounds have been preserved. Enjoy the view from the top of the lighthouse and also the interpretive information about the lighthouse keepers. They lived with their families at this solitary outpost, helping ships avoid the offshore shoals between Savannah and Charleston. Other park visitors will be surf fishing or angling from the 1,120-foot pier extending into Fripp Island Inlet, in hopes of catching whiting, speckle trout, drum, or flounder.

You can enjoy the beautiful forest via the 8 miles of trails that course through the park's interior. One trail leads from the campground access road to the historic lighthouse area. Another path makes a 6-mile loop to the end of the island by the fishing pier and back. The mainland side of the park features a boardwalk through an estuarine marsh and also has a wildlife viewing area. The most appealing aspect of the park is its pristine natural state and lack of commercialism and high-rise condos. During busy times, the campground itself can seem bustling, but not compared with other beach destinations. Spring and fall are ideal times to enjoy this park, but any time is better than no time at all.

MAP

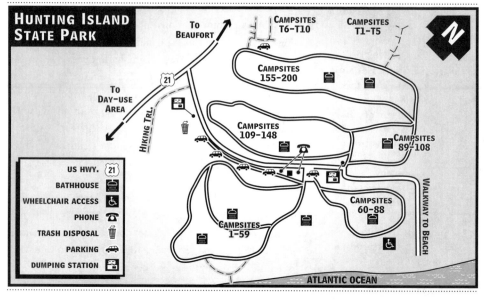

HUNTING ISLAND STATE PARK

To BEAUFORT

CAMPSITES T6-T10

CAMPSITES T1-T5

To DAY-USE AREA

21

CAMPSITES 155-200

HIKING TRL.

CAMPSITES 109-148

CAMPSITES 89-108

CAMPSITES 60-88

CAMPSITES 1-59

WALKWAY TO BEACH

ATLANTIC OCEAN

US HWY. 21
BATHHOUSE
WHEELCHAIR ACCESS
PHONE
TRASH DISPOSAL
PARKING
DUMPING STATION

GETTING THERE

From Exit 33 on I-95, take US 21 south 42 miles, through the town of Beaufort and staying with US 21 to Hunting Island. Turn left on Campground Road to reach the campground.

GPS COORDINATES

UTM Zone (WGS84) 17S
Easting 0553140
Northing 3582600
Latitude 32 22' 51.3"
Longitude 80 26' 6.0"

> *This oceanside park is close—but not too close— to Myrtle Beach.*

CAMPERS COME TO HUNTINGTON BEACH for a variety of reasons. Many enjoy the beach and other natural aspects of this 2,500-acre preserve in a fast-developing coast. Others relax in the campground after seeking activities outside the park. Either way, they enjoy this getaway, one of the limited public-beach camping locales in South Carolina. This one has the added benefit—or detraction, depending on how you look at it—of being 16 miles from the heart of Myrtle Beach.

The campground, a short walk from the beach, has two large loops with a separate walk-in tent-camping area. The first loop has the sites closest to the beach, in a mix of sun and shade from planted cedars and live oaks. This is the land of the RV, but there are some good sites here. Make reservations for odd-numbered sites 1 through 31 in this loop. A recreation building, near site 19, is convenient for getting out of those inevitable summer thunderstorms. Avoid sites 74 through 88 and 90 through 102, which are located on crossroads within the loop. Most sites on the remainder of the first loop have at least one shade tree. (Woe to those stuck in a sunny site on a hot South Carolina summer day.) The second loop has the sites farthest from the ocean. Many of them have thick brush between sites, offering good privacy but little overhead shade.

Try to get one of the walk-in tent sites if you can; they are first come, first served. To reach them, leave the walk-in parking area and follow a sandy trail past a water spigot. Site T-1 lies beneath a large live oak. T-2 is more open. T-3 is shaded by pines and live oaks. T-4 is rather small. T-5 is large and well shaded. T-6 is the farthest back and set amid privacy-giving brush.

This popular state park fills weekends from March to September and many weekdays during the peak of summer. Many sites can be reserved, especially those

RATINGS

Beauty: ☆ ☆ ☆
Privacy: ☆ ☆ ☆
Spaciousness: ☆ ☆ ☆
Quiet: ☆ ☆ ☆ ☆
Security: ☆ ☆ ☆ ☆ ☆
Cleanliness: ☆ ☆ ☆

closest to the beach. These beachside sites are often filled with RVs—location has its price, but proximity to an ocean breeze will cut down on insects when they are bothersome (usually following rainy periods). The walk-in tent sites offer much more privacy and the experience tent campers are after. A camp store is conveniently located inside the park.

Huntington Beach State Park prides itself on its naturalist programs. Checking out the alligators on the park causeway is a popular pastime. Let park personnel inform you about these ancient creatures. Other programs cover birding, the salt marsh, seashells, whales, dolphins, and the historic homesite known as Atalaya. This winter home of park benefactors Collis and Anna Huntington is modeled after houses on the Spanish Mediterranean coast. Rangers lead tours of this home, and three different park programs are held during the busy season, March through September. The park education center offers more learning experiences.

Three miles of beachfront attract ocean enthusiasts who shell, surf fish, or just relax while listening to the waves roll in. I first came here more than two decades ago. A jetty at the north end of the beach is also a popular fishing spot. Some folks will be hiking the two nature trails or kayaking the saltwater marsh. But many others will be enjoying the attractions of the nearby tourist destinations at Myrtle Beach, ranging from miniature golf to dinner shows to waterslides. Shoppers will be looking for the perfect grass basket from the area or a hammock from Pawleys Island. So whether you prefer to shop and act the part of the hokey tourist or to just enjoy the undeveloped shoreline, Huntington Beach may be the place for you.

KEY INFORMATION

ADDRESS: 16148 Ocean Hwy. Murrells Inlet, SC 29576

OPERATED BY: South Carolina State Parks

INFORMATION: (843) 237-4440; southcarolina parks.com; reservations: (866) 345-7275, reserve america.com

OPEN: Year-round

SITES: 6 walk-in tent sites, 133 others

EACH SITE: Walk-in sites have picnic table, fire ring; 123 sites have water and electricity; 10 sites also have sewer

ASSIGNMENT: First come, first served and by reservation

REGISTRATION: At office–gift shop

FACILITIES: Hot showers, flush toilets, water spigots

PARKING: At campsites and at walk-in tent-camping parking area

FEE: $17–$19 tent sites, $25–$28 other sites, depending on season

ELEVATION: Sea level

RESTRICTIONS: *Pets:* On leash only *Fires:* In fire rings only *Alcohol:* Prohibited *Vehicles:* None *Other:* 14-day stay limit

MAP

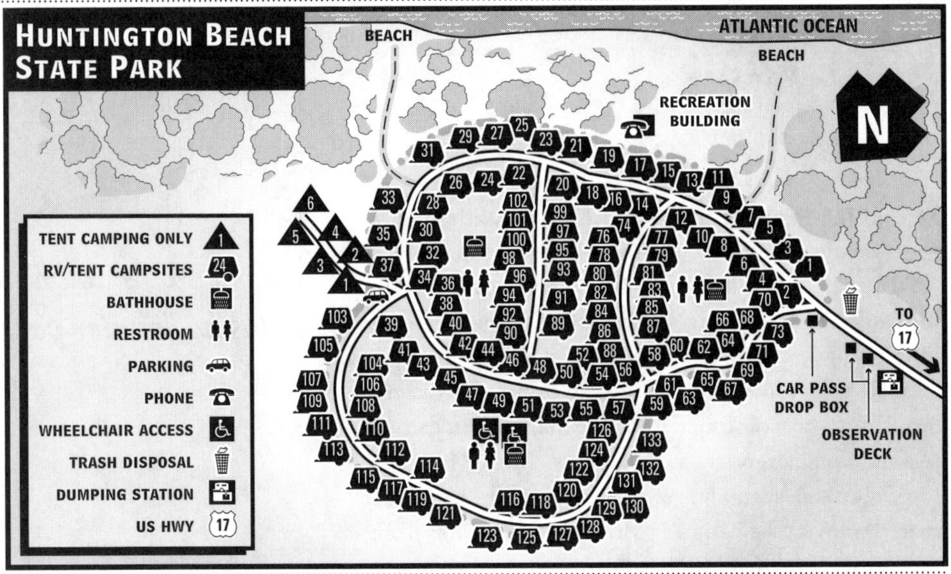

HUNTINGTON BEACH STATE PARK

ATLANTIC OCEAN

BEACH

BEACH

RECREATION BUILDING

N

TENT CAMPING ONLY	
RV/TENT CAMPSITES	
BATHHOUSE	
RESTROOM	
PARKING	
PHONE	
WHEELCHAIR ACCESS	
TRASH DISPOSAL	
DUMPING STATION	
US HWY	17

CAR PASS DROP BOX

OBSERVATION DECK

TO 17

GETTING THERE

From Myrtle Beach, take US 17 south 16 miles to the state park, on your left.

GPS COORDINATES

UTM Zone (WGS84) 17S
Easting 0679840
Northing 3708880
Latitude 33 30' 22.2"
Longitude 79 3' 50.4"

L **ITTLE PEE DEE STATE PARK** is one of those destinations that time seems to have passed by. The park exudes an atmosphere as slow moving as the Little Pee Dee River, for which it is named. I drove in during a weekday and barely saw a soul, other than a ranger who rolled by after I set up camp. After registering me, he confirmed that the park is indeed as relaxing and forgotten as it appears. In his 12 years there, he had seen the 52-site campground fill only twice. Many of the campers who do visit are folks from the Myrtle Beach area who want to escape the madness that sometimes envelops that tourist destination.

Time slows down at this backwater park.

The campground is laid out in a grand loop along the shores of Lake Norton. The sandy road leads to sand parking spurs. Many pines and oaks grow overhead, while dogwoods are a prevalent understory tree. Oddly, the first two campsites in the loop are 49 and 50. Then the numbering becomes more conventional. Two small subloops spur from the main loop. Curve toward the lake, passing a picnic area with a covered shelter near site 7 and pass some lakeside sites. Large and well separated from each other, these sites have raked-sand floors, with needles and oak leaves marking their perimeter. Because the campground rarely gets crowded, you likely won't have a neighbor at the campsite next door, so privacy isn't much of an issue.

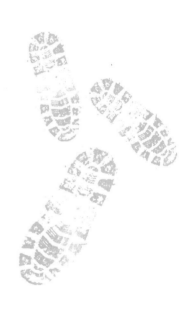

The subloop curves away from the lake and joins the main loop; lakeside sites resume with site 20. The next few sites, which offer great vistas of Lake Norton, are the campground's most coveted. Leaving the lake again, the official tent sites start with site 33. Because they are nonelectric, they are cheaper and in less demand than the electric sites.

I stayed in site 34 and was the only tent camper that night, warmed by a piney fire. A front moved in later, further warming the air and bringing rain. Breaking camp

RATINGS

Beauty: ✰ ✰ ✰
Privacy: ✰ ✰ ✰
Spaciousness: ✰ ✰ ✰ ✰
Quiet: ✰ ✰ ✰ ✰
Security: ✰ ✰ ✰ ✰ ✰
Cleanliness: ✰ ✰ ✰ ✰

ADDRESS: 1298 State Park Rd. Dillon, SC 29536

OPERATED BY: South Carolina State Parks

INFORMATION: (843) 774-8872; southcarolina parks.com; reservations: (866) 345-7275, reserve america.com

OPEN: Year-round

SITES: 18 tent sites, 32 other sites

EACH SITE: Tent sites have picnic tables, fire rings, water

ASSIGNMENT: First come, first served and by reservation

REGISTRATION: Ranger will come by to register you

FACILITIES: Hot showers, flush toilets

PARKING: At campsites only

FEE: $9–$10 tent sites, $12–$13 others

ELEVATION: 100 feet

RESTRICTIONS: *Pets:* On leash only
Fires: In fire rings only
Alcohol: Prohibited
Vehicles: None
Other: 14-day stay limit

in the rain is never fun, but it's a fact of tent camping if you do it often enough.

The Beaver Pond Nature Trail begins just past site 40. This is more of a leg-stretching path than a bona fide hiking trail, though it does loop to a beaver pond. The tent sites here have thicker woods around them, are less used, and angle ever so slightly downhill toward Lake Norton. Complete the loop near some very large tent sites suitable for a family gathering. At the center of the loop are two bathhouses, the newer of which is heated, a fact I appreciated during my late-fall trip. A play area is also in the loop's center.

This part of South Carolina, Dillon County, is rural and relaxing. Little Pee Dee's 835 acres, stretched along the Little Pee Dee River, mark the apex of this quietness. A park lake, adding more aquatic beauty, complements the river and adjoining swamp. The damming of Bell Swamp Branch and Indian Pot Branch forms Lake Norton. The 54-acre impoundment is a no-gas-motors lake, keeping the atmosphere serene. It does have a boat launch, however, and offers boat rentals for those who want to tour the lake or do some freshwater fishing. Anglers can also fish from the banks of the lake or from the nearby lake dam.

The park's namesake is also a boating possibility. The Little Pee Dee is a fine example of a coastal-plain blackwater river. Cypress trees and tupelo line much of it, as do sandbars, which are great for picnicking or relaxing. The river is tough to access from the park bridge but boasts landings and accesses nearby. Instead of trying to figure out all the particulars of a canoe trip, though, why not leave it to the outfitters? Betwixt the Rivers, based in nearby Marion, South Carolina, offers trips of varying lengths. Reach them at (843) 423-1919. Make sure you have a little extra time on your hands, as life is slow and relaxing in this part of the Palmetto State.

MAP

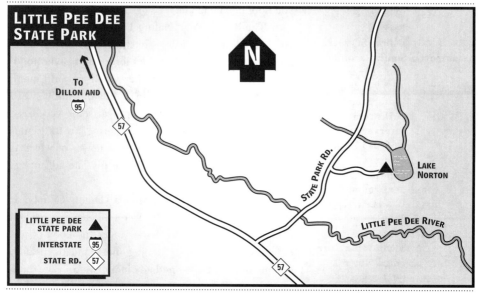

From Exit 193 on I-95 near
Dillon, take SC 57 south as it
twists and turns through
Dillon, and stay with SC 57
11.2 miles from the interstate, to reach State Park
Road. Turn left on State Park
Road, and follow it 2 miles
to the state park entrance,
on your right.

GPS COORDINATES

UTM Zone (WGS84) 17S
Easting 0650320
Northing 3799820
Latitude 34 20' 49.4"
Longitude 79 10' 16.2"

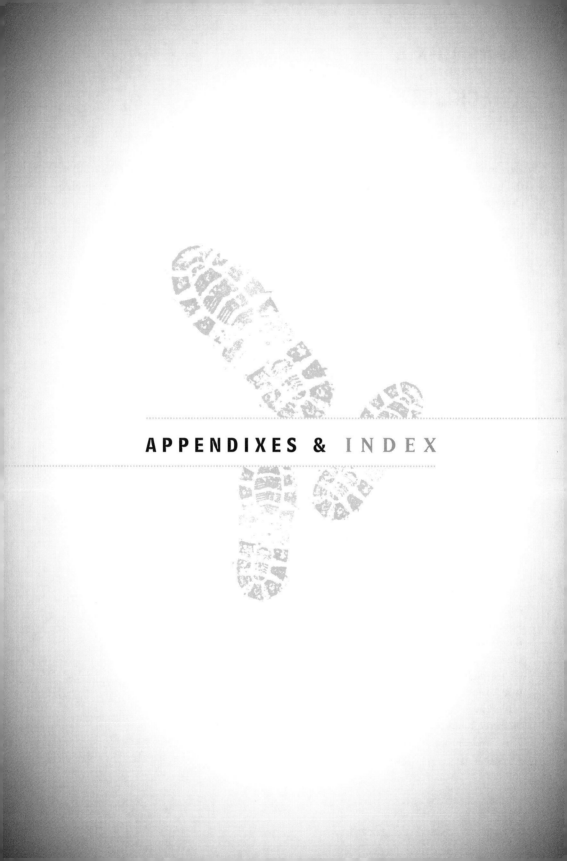

APPENDIXES & INDEX

APPENDIX A
CAMPING-EQUIPMENT CHECKLIST

Except for the large and bulky items on this list, I keep a plastic storage container full of the essentials of car camping so that they're ready to go when I am. I make a last-minute check of the inventory, resupply anything that's low or missing, and away I go!

COOKING UTENSILS

Bottle opener
Bottles of salt, pepper, spices, and sugar
Can opener
Cooking oil and maple syrup in
    water-proof, spillproof containers
Corkscrew
Cups, plastic or tin
Dish soap (biodegradable), sponge, towel
Fire starter
Flatware
Food of your choice
Frying pan, spatula
Fuel for stove
Lighter, matches in waterproof container
Plates
Pocketknife
Pot with lid
Stove
Tinfoil
Wooden spoon

FIRST-AID KIT

Antibiotic cream
Aspirin or ibuprofen
Band-Aids
Diphenhydramine (Benadryl)
Gauze pads
Insect repellent
Moleskin
Sunscreen and lip balm
Tape, waterproof adhesive
Tweezers

SLEEPING GEAR

Pillow
Sleeping bag
Sleeping pad, inflatable or insulated
Tent with ground sheet and rainfly

MISCELLANEOUS

Bath soap (biodegradable), washcloth,
    and towel
Camp chair
Candles
Cooler
Deck of cards
Flashlight or headlamp
Lantern
Maps (road, trail, topographic,
    and the like)
Paper towels
Sunglasses
Toilet paper
Water bottle
Weather radio
Wool blanket
Zip-top plastic bags

OPTIONAL

Barbecue grill
Binoculars
Field guides on bird, plant, and wildlife
    identification
Fishing rod and tackle
Hatchet

APPENDIX B
SOURCES
OF INFORMATION

The following is a partial list of agencies, associations, and organizations to write or call for information on outdoor recreation opportunities in the Carolinas.

NORTH CAROLINA

North Carolina Great Smoky Mountains National Park
107 Park Headquarters Road
Gatlinburg, TN 37320
(865) 436-1200; **nps.gov/grsm**

National Forests in North Carolina
160A Zillicoa Street
P.O. Box 2750
Asheville, NC 28802
(828) 257-4200; **cs.unca.edu/nfsnc**

Blue Ridge Parkway
199 Hemphill Knob Road
Asheville, NC 28803
(828) 271-4779; **nps.gov/blri**

North Carolina Department of Tourism
301 North Wilmington Street
Raleigh, NC 27601
(800) VISIT-NC (847-4862)
visitnc.com

North Carolina State Parks
1615 MSC
Raleigh, NC 27699
(919) 733-PARK (7275)
ncparks.gov

SOUTH CAROLINA

Francis Marion and Sumter National Forest
4931 Broad River Road
Columbia, SC 29212
(828) 257-4200; **fs.fed.us/r8/fms**

Kings Mountain National Military Park
2625 Park Road
Blacksburg, SC 29702
(864) 936-7921; **nps.gov/kimo**

South Carolina Department of Tourism
1205 Pendleton Street
Columbia, SC 29201
(803) 734-1062
discoversouthcarolina.com

South Carolina State Parks
1205 Pendleton Street
Columbia, SC 29201
(888) 88-PARKS (887-2757)
southcarolinaparks.com

U.S. Army Corps of Engineers
U.S. Army Corps of Engineers
Savannah District
P.O. Box 889
Savannah, GA 40201
(912) 652-5822; **sas.usace.army.mil**

INDEX

THE BEST
IN TENT
CAMPING
CAROLINAS

ABOUT THE AUTHOR

Johnny Molloy is an outdoor writer based in Johnson City, Tennessee. Born in Memphis, he moved to Knoxville in 1980 to attend the University of Tennessee. It was there in Knoxville that he developed his love of the natural world that has since become the primary focus of his life.

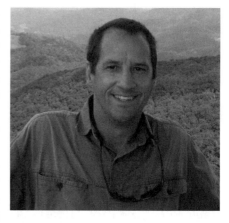

It all started on a backpacking foray into the Great Smoky Mountains National Park.

That first trip, though a disaster, unleashed an innate love of the outdoors that has led to his spending more than 110 nights in the wild per year over the past 25 years, backpacking and canoe camping throughout our country and abroad. In 1987, after graduating from the University of Tennessee with a degree in economics, he continued to spend an ever-increasing amount of time in natural places, becoming more skilled in a variety of environments. Friends enjoyed his adventure stories; one even suggested he write a book. Soon he parlayed his love of the outdoors into an occupation.

The results of his efforts are more than 30 books, ranging from hiking guides to paddling guides, to camping guides, and true-outdoor-adventure stories. His books primarily cover the Southeast but range to Colorado and Wisconsin. Carolina books of Molloy's include *Day and Overnight Hikes: the Great Smoky Mountains National Park* and *50 Hikes in South Carolina*.

Molloy has also written numerous articles for magazines such as *Backpacker* and *Sea Kayaker,* and for Web sites such as gorp.com. He continues to write and travel extensively to all four corners of the United States, endeavoring in a variety of outdoor pursuits. For the latest information about Molloy, visit **johnnymolloy.com.**

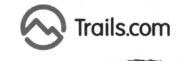
Day & Overnight Hikes: Great Smoky Mountains National Park

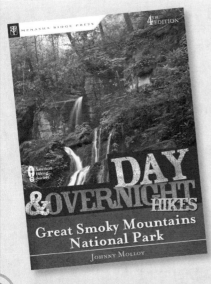

by Johnny Molloy
ISBN: 978-0-89732-662-9
4th Edition, 5x7, paperback, $13.95
224 pages, maps, photographs, index

The Great Smoky Mountains National Park is the most visited of America's national parks. With 500,000 acres of land and over nine million visitors annually, discovering the beauty and solitude of this national park can be difficult. This update of the popular *Day and Overnight Hikes Great Smoky Mountains National Park,* with a new cover and trim size, is the definitive guide for the novice and veteran hiker alike. All of the information needed to confidently hit the trail is in this comprehensive and compact guide. Each profile includes significant sites along the way.

 MENASHA RIDGE PRESS
 www.menasharidge.com

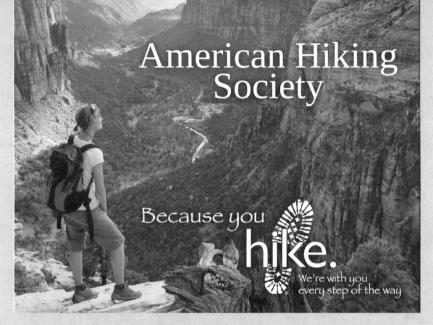

American Hiking Society

Because you hike.
We're with you every step of the way

Since its founding in 1976, **American Hiking Society** has been the only national voice for hikers—dedicated to promoting and protecting America's hiking trails, their surrounding natural areas and the hiking experience. **American Hiking Society** works every day:

- Speaking for hikers in the halls of Congress and with federal land managers
- Building and maintaining hiking trails
- Educating and supporting hikers by providing information and resources
- Supporting hiking and trail organizations nationwide

Whether you're a casual hiker or a seasoned backpacker, become a member of **American Hiking Society** and join the national hiking community! You'll not only enjoy great members-only benefits but you will help ensure the hiking trails you love will remain protected and will be waiting for you the next time you lace up your boots and hit the trail.

We invite you to join us today!

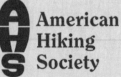

American Hiking Society

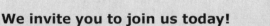

1422 Fenwick Lane · Silver Spring, MD 20910 · (800) 972-8608
www.AmericanHiking.org · info@AmericanHiking.org

DEAR CUSTOMERS AND FRIENDS,

SUPPORTING YOUR INTEREST IN OUTDOOR ADVENTURE, travel, and an active lifestyle is central to our operations, from the authors we choose to the locations we detail to the way we design our books. Menasha Ridge Press was incorporated in 1982 by a group of veteran outdoorsmen and professional outfitters. For 25 years now, we've specialized in creating books that benefit the outdoors enthusiast.

Almost immediately, Menasha Ridge Press earned a reputation for revolutionizing outdoors- and travel-guidebook publishing. For such activities as canoeing, kayaking, hiking, backpacking, and mountain biking, we established new standards of quality that transformed the whole genre, resulting in outdoor-recreation guides of great sophistication and solid content. Menasha Ridge continues to be outdoor publishing's greatest innovator.

The folks at Menasha Ridge Press are as at home on a white-water river or mountain trail as they are editing a manuscript. The books we build for you are the best they can be, because we're responding to your needs. Plus, we use and depend on them ourselves.

We look forward to seeing you on the river or the trail. If you'd like to contact us directly, join in at www.trekalong.com or visit us at www.menasharidge.com. We thank you for your interest in our books and the natural world around us all.

SAFE TRAVELS,

Bob Sehlinger

BOB SEHLINGER
PUBLISHER

MAP LEGEND

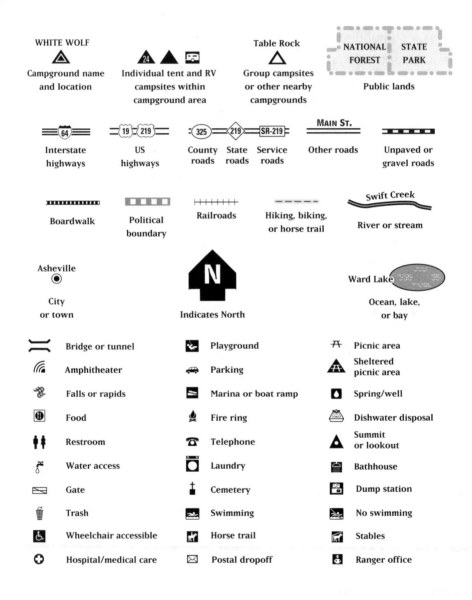

WHITE WOLF

Campground name
and location

Individual tent and RV
campsites within
campground area

Table Rock

Group campsites
or other nearby
campgrounds

NATIONAL   STATE
FOREST   PARK

Public lands

64
Interstate
highways

19 219
US
highways

325 219 SR-219
County State Service
roads   roads roads

MAIN ST.
Other roads

Unpaved or
gravel roads

Boardwalk

Political
boundary

Railroads

Hiking, biking,
or horse trail

Swift Creek
River or stream

Asheville

City
or town

N

Indicates North

Ward Lake

Ocean, lake,
or bay

Bridge or tunnel	Playground	Picnic area
Amphitheater	Parking	Sheltered picnic area
Falls or rapids	Marina or boat ramp	Spring/well
Food	Fire ring	Dishwater disposal
Restroom	Telephone	Summit or lookout
Water access	Laundry	Bathhouse
Gate	Cemetery	Dump station
Trash	Swimming	No swimming
Wheelchair accessible	Horse trail	Stables
Hospital/medical care	Postal dropoff	Ranger office

THE BEST
IN TENT
CAMPING
CAROLINAS